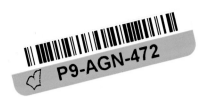

CLINICAL PSYCHOPHARMACOLOGY

**made
ridiculously
simple**

John Preston, Psy.D., ABPP
Alliant International University
Sacramento, California

James Johnson, M.D.
Kaiser Medical Center
Department of Psychiatry
South Sacramento, California

ISBN #0-940780-44-5

Made in the United States of America

Published by
MedMaster, Inc.
P.O. Box 640028
Miami, Fla. 33164

For Bonnie and Mary

Contents

Preface

This brief book provides an overview of clinical psychopharmacology. Successful medical treatment of emotional and mental disorders depends on two factors: a thorough knowledge of psychotropic medications and an accurate diagnosis. Both issues are addressed in this book in a practical and concise format.

To the best of our knowledge, recommended doses for medications listed in this book are accurate. However, they are not meant to serve as a guide for prescription of medications. Please check the manufacturer's product information sheet or the *Physicians' Desk Reference* for any changes in dosage schedule or contraindications.

We wish to express our appreciation to the following people who have reviewed this book and made a number of helpful suggestions: John H. Greist, M.D., Donald Klein, M.D., Glen Hakanson, M.D., and Patrick Donlon, M.D. Many thanks to Michelle Riekstins for her help in the preparation of the manuscript and to our editor, Dr. Stephen Goldberg, for many helpful suggestions.

Chapter 1   General Principles

BIOLOGY vs. PSYCHOLOGY

For many years a debate raged in psychiatry with regard to the etiology and treatment of major mental disorders. Two opposing camps emerged: biological psychiatry, whose devotees held that psychiatric disorders had an organic basis; and psychologically oriented psychiatry, probably best represented by the psychodynamic movement, whose converts focused on the role of current emotional stressors, early childhood traumas, interpersonal problems, and intrapsychic conflict as causal agents in the development of psychiatric symptomatology. Although these polar views still exist, in recent years there has been an emerging view that encompasses both psychological and physiological factors in the etiology and treatment of many psychiatric disorders. In many, if not most, mental disorders it is helpful to think of a continuum or spectrum. Almost all mental disorders usually represent heterogeneous syndromes.

When one talks about depression, for instance, it is important to realize that depression can present in a number of different ways and may have diverse etiologies. In some instances the cause may be purely psychological, e.g., a reaction to losing a job, death of a loved one, a significant rejection, etc. Likewise, symptoms may be largely psychological, e.g., feelings of low self-esteem and sadness. In other cases the picture is one of a pure biological disorder which has little or no connection to environmental precipitants, but rather involves an endogenous neurochemical malfunction. In addition to psychological symptoms, the resulting symptoms may include a host of somatic symptoms, such as sleep disturbance and weight loss. Clearly, in some individuals there is an interplay of environmental/psychological factors *and* biochemical dysfunctions. The question "Is this a psychological or biological problem?" is overly simplistic. Rather, one must ask, "To what extent is this disorder due to psychological factors and to what extent is it due to a biochemical disturbance?" The answer to this question is extremely important in guiding treatment decisions. *Most purely psychological problems are not helped by medication treatment. On the other hand, most biologically based psychiatric disorders require medication treatment.*

In this book we hope to provide key diagnostic guidelines to help the clinician pinpoint the diagnosis and develop a realistic treatment plan.

Chapter 2   Depression

DIAGNOSIS

Major Clinical Features and Differential Diagnosis

It is important to distinguish between (1) reactive sadness, (2) grief, (3) medical illness and medications that cause depressive symptoms, and (4) clinical depression. The first two are painful but normal emotional reactions and usually do not require treatment. These four syndromes may be distinguished by the following characteristics:

1. *Reactive Sadness.* The emotional reaction stems from a relatively minor event. It is transient (a few hours to a few days) and rarely interferes with functioning.

2. *Grief.* This is a normal response to a major interpersonal loss (such as the death of a loved one or marital separation/divorce). This process can be tremendously painful and is much more prolonged than reactive sadness. Grief differs from clinical depression in three ways:

   a. Despite intense sadness, there is no significant loss of self-esteem.

   b. The patient clearly relates the sadness to the loss. There may be active mourning and pining for the loved one; the painful feelings "make sense."

   c. Grief work (i.e., mourning) and time are often the major ingredients necessary for emotional healing.
   Note that at least 25% of people experiencing a major loss will initially exhibit grief reactions, but during the year following the loss will go on to develop major depression. Additionally, 10% of bereaved individuals will develop traumatic stress symptoms following interpersonal losses (e.g. intense anxiety, nightmares). Thus one must have a high index of suspicion for these common forms of complicated bereavement.

3. *Medical Illnesses and Medications That Can Cause Depression.* Certain medical disorders (see Figure 1) can at times result in biochemical changes that affect central neurotransmitters, thereby triggering serious depressive reactions. Likewise, some medications can cause depression as a side effect (see Figure 2). Please note that minor tranquilizers may cause or exacerbate depression. A very frequent treatment mistake is for the physician to be impressed by the more obvious symptoms of anxiety or agitation, to fail to recognize an underlying depression, and to prescribe a benzodiazepine/minor tranquilizer. The result is often some initial calming, but after a few weeks the depression worsens. If the basic disorder is depression, but with coexisting anxiety symptoms, it is impor-

tant to treat the depression. With appropriate treatment for the depression, the anxiety symptoms will generally subside.

When the basic cause of depression is one of the illnesses listed in Figure 1 or a side effect of medication, the primary focus should be on treating the core illness or switching medications. When such interventions are carried out, the depression will usually lift.

Figure 1

COMMON DISORDERS THAT MAY CAUSE DEPRESSION

- Addison's disease
- AIDS
- Anemia
- Apnea
- Asthma
- Chronic Fatigue Syndromes
- Chronic infection (mononucleosis, TB)
- Chronic pain
- Congestive heart failure
- Cushing's disease
- Diabetes
- Hyperthyroidism
- Hypothyroidism
- Infectious Hepatitis
- Influenza
- Malignancies (cancer)
- Malnutrition
- Menopause
- Multiple sclerosis
- Parkinson's disease
- Post-partum hormonal changes
- Porphyria
- Premenstrual syndrome
- Rheumatoid arthritis
- Syphilis
- Systemic lupus erythematosis
- Ulcerative colitis
- Uremia

4. *Clinical Depression.* This is a pathological process characterized as follows:

   a. Depressed mood (sadness or emptiness) or irritability is often continuous and pervasive.

   b. A loss of interest in normal life activities.

   c. There is increasing impairment of normal functioning (work, school, and intimate relationships).

   d. There is an irrational or exaggerated erosion of self-esteem.

   e. There is a dramatic and specific change in vegetative patterns (e.g., sleep, appetite, sex drive, etc.) and the appearance of nonspecific physical complaints.

   f. Depression can occur in response to psychological stressors, or may emerge without clear-cut precipitating events.

Figure 2

DRUGS THAT MAY CAUSE DEPRESSION

TYPE	GENERIC NAME	BRAND NAME
Antihypertensives (for high blood pressure)	reserpine	Serpasil, Ser-Ap-Es, Sandril
	propranolol hydrochloride	Inderal
	methyldopa	Aldomet
	guanethidine sulfate	Ismelin sulfate
	clonidine hydrochloride	Catapres
	hydralazine hydrochloride	Apresoline hydrochloride
Corticosteroids and other Hormones	cortisone acetate	Cortone
	estrogen	Evex, Menrium, Femest
	progesterone and derivatives	Lipo-Lutin, Progestasert, Proluton
Antiparkinson Drugs	levodopa and carbidopa	Sinemet
	levodopa	Dopar, Larodopa
	amantadine hydrochloride	Symmetrel
Antianxiety Drugs	diazepam and others	Valium (see Figure 21)
Birth Control Pills	progesterone estrogen	Various Brands
Alcohol	wine, beer, spirits	Various Brands

Target Symptoms

All types of depression tend to share certain universal symptoms (see Figure 3). Disorders that reflect an underlying biochemical dysfunction typically present with *both* the universal symptoms *and* the physiological symptoms, listed below: (See Figure 4).

ANTIDEPRESSANT MEDICATION

When Do You Prescribe Antidepressants?

The most important guideline for prescribing antidepressant medication is whether or not there are sustained physiological symptoms, as outlined below (see Figure 4). Occasional disturbances of sleep or appetite, for instance, do not

Figure 3

SYMPTOMS COMMON TO ALL DEPRESSIONS

- Mood of sadness, despair, emptiness
- Anhedonia (loss of the ability to experience pleasure)[1]
- Low self-esteem
- Apathy, low motivation, and social withdrawal
- Excessive emotional sensitivity
- Negative, pessimistic thinking
- Irritability and low frustration tolerance
- Suicidal ideas

---

[1]*Note:* Some degree of decreased capacity for pleasure may be seen in all types of depression. In depressions that involve a biochemical disturbance, this loss of ability to experience pleasure can become so pronounced that the patient has almost no moments of joy or pleasure. Such people are said to have a "non-reactive mood," which means that they are unable to temporarily get out of their depressed mood.

Figure 4

VEGETATIVE/PHYSIOLOGICAL SYMPTOMS REFLECTING A BIOCHEMICAL DYSFUNCTION
(TARGET SYMPTOMS FOR MEDICATION TREATMENT)

- Sleep disturbance (early morning awakening, decreased sleep efficiency, frequent awakenings throughout the night,[1] occasionally hypersomnia: excessive sleeping)
- Appetite disturbance (decreased or increased, with accompanying weight loss or gain)
- Fatigue
- Decreased sex drive
- Restlessness, agitation, or psychomotor retardation
- Diurnal variations in mood (usually feeling worse in the morning)
- Impaired concentration and forgetfulness
- Pronounced anhedonia (total loss of the ability to experience pleasure)

---

[1]*Note:* Initial insomnia (difficulty in falling asleep) may be seen with depression but is not diagnostic of a major depressive disorder. Initial insomnia can be seen in anyone experiencing stress in general. Initial insomnia alone is more characteristic of anxiety disorders than of depression.

warrant medication treatment. However, if there is continuing weight loss, marked fatigue each day, and poor sleep most nights, antidepressants are indicated. In the Appendix we have included a brief symptom checklist that can be used to quickly assess a host of psychiatric symptoms. Depressive symptoms are included under Section A. Additionally, those patients who are depressed and are judged to be poor psychotherapy candidates (e.g., lower intelligence, not psychologically minded, or refuse psychotherapy) should be considered for a trial on antidepressants.

Choosing Medication

Antidepressant medications fall into two primary groups: (1) typical antidepressants, and (2) MAO inhibitors. Emperical studies suggest that certain symptomatic presentations may point toward preferred first-line medication choices. This has resulted in the development of treatment guidelines. If the clinical picture is dominated by: anxiety, agitation, obsessional symptoms, rumination, irritability, aggression, and/or pronounced suicidality, serotonin reuptake inhibitors are the first line treatment strategy (see Figure 10). If the clinical picture is characterized by: apathy, low energy, anhedonia, and/or low motivation, noradrenergic reuptake blockers are preferred (e.g. bupropion).

A second major factor in choosing an antidepressant is the side effect profile (side effects are described below).

Prescribing Treatment

Antidepressant medications are generally started at a low dosage and gradually titrated up. The most common mistake made by family physicians is to under-medicate. Although there are exceptions, generally a patient (ages 16–55) must receive a dose that is within the therapeutic range (see Figure 5). (Doses for those over 55 are often somewhat lower.)

Typical start-up regimes would be as follows:

Drug	(doses for adults ages 16-55) Starting dose	Increase in 1-2 weeks, if tolerated
Fluoxetine	10 mg	20 mg
Sertaline	50 mg	100 mg
Paroxetine	10 mg	20 mg
Citalopram	20 mg	40 mg
Venlafaxine, XR	37.5 mg	75 mg
Bupropion, SR	100 mg	100 mg bid
Nefazodone	50 mg bid	100 mg bid
Mirtazapine	15 mg	30 mg
Escitalopram	5 mg	10 mg

Increases in dose can be made if there is a failure to show a positive response after 4–5 weeks of treatment. Note: If patient had first episode prior to 18, is experiencing a recurrent episode, and/or has been depressed for more than two months, often requires 4–6 weeks to show first signs of clinical response.

Figure 5

ANTIDEPRESSANT MEDICATIONS

| NAMES | | USUAL DAILY DOSAGE | | ACH |
GENERIC	BRAND	RANGE	SEDATION	EFFECTS[1]
TYPICAL ANTIDEPRESSANTS				
imipramine	Tofranil	150–300 mg	mid	mid
desipramine	Norpramin	150–300 mg	low	low
amitriptyline	Elavil	150–300 mg	high	high
nortriptyline	Aventyl, Pamelor	75–125 mg	mid	mid
protriptyline	Vivactil	15–40 mg	low	mid
trimipramine	Surmontil	100–300 mg	high	mid
doxepin	Sinequan, Adapin	150–300 mg	high	mid
maprotiline	Ludiomil	150–225 mg	mid	low
amoxapine	Asendin	150–400 mg	mid	low
trazodone	Desyrel[2]	150–400 mg	mid	none
fluoxetine*	Prozac, Sarafem	20–80 mg	low	none
bupropion, S.R.	Wellbutrin, S.R.	150–300 mg	low	none
sertraline*	Zoloft	50–200 mg	low	none
paroxetine*	Paxil	20–50 mg	low	low
venlafaxine, X.R.	Effexor, X.R.	75–350 mg	low	none
nefazodone	Serzone[2]	100–500 mg	mid	low
fluvoxamine*	Luvox	50–300 mg	low	low
mirtazapine	Remeron	15–45 mg	mid	mid
citalopram*	Celexa	10–60 mg	low	none
escitalopram*	Lexapro	5–20 mg	low	none
reboxetine	Vestra	4–8 mg	low	none
MAO INHIBITORS[3]				
phenelzine	Nardil	30–90 mg	low	none
tranylcypromine	Parnate	20–60 mg	low	none
isocarboxazid	Marplan	10–40 mg	low	none

[1]*ACH EFFECTS* (anticholinergic side effects) include dry mouth, constipation, difficulty in urinating, and blurry vision. Can cause confusion and memory disturbances in the elderly or brain damaged patient.

[2]Due to short half-life, requires divided dosing.

[3]Require strict adherence to dietary and medication regimen.

Note: prescribe maprotiline and bupropion to patients with history of seizures only with great caution.

*A widely prescribed class of antidepressants are the *selective serotonin reuptake inhibitors* (SSRIs), which include: fluoxetine, paroxetine, sertraline, fluvoxamine, citalopram, and escitalopram.

Figure 6

DECISION TREE FOR DIAGNOSIS
AND TREATMENT OF DEPRESSION - I

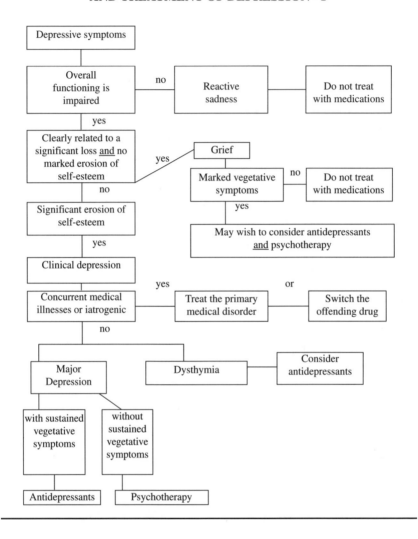

The treatment of major depression involves three phases:

Acute Treatment: Begins with the first dose and extends until the patient is asymptomatic (in good case scenarios, this may be from 6–8 weeks).

Continuation Treatment: To avoid acute relapse, it is strongly suggested that patients continue treatment for a minimum of six months beyond the acute phase.

Figure 6 (cont.)

DECISION TREE: TREATMENT OF DEPRESSION - II

Phase of Treatment

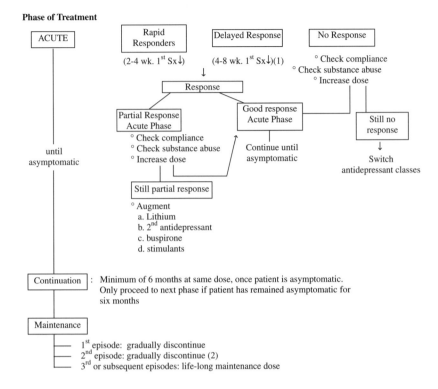

Footnotes:
1. Patients with the following characteristics may ultimately be good responders, but take longer to achieve first signs of symptomatic improvement: current episode has been ongoing for more than three months and the symptoms are severe.
2. If a second episode and these risk factors are present, may consider life-long treatment: first episode was prior to the age of 18, family history of mood disorders, inter-episode the patient was not euthymic (i.e. did not fully recover from first episode).
3. This decision tree is based on results from the Texas Medication Algorithm Project (1998) and A. John Rush (1997). Note that the general concepts from the project are addressed in this decision tree, however the particular graphics above were developed by the authors of this book.

Also, recent studies indicate that the patient should be maintained on the *same* dose used during the acute phase.

Maintenance Treatment: Relapse prevention is an important aspect of treatment, especially in those patients judged to have recurrent episodes (or at risk for

Figure 7

SPECIAL PROBLEMS AND MEDICATIONS OF CHOICE

THE PROBLEM	DRUGS OF CHOICE
1. High suicide risk[1]	1. trazodone, SSRIs, bupropion, venlafaxine
2. Concurrent depression and panic attacks	2. phenelzine, imipramine, SSRIs
3. Chronic pain with or without depression	3. amitriptyline, doxepin, venlafaxine
4. Weight gain on other antidepressants	4. bupropion, SSRIs[2]
5. Sensitivity to anticholinergic side effects	5. trazodone, phenelzine, tranylcypromine, bupropion, SSRIs (except paroxetine)
6. Orthostatic hypotension	6. nortriptyline, bupropion, sertraline
7. Sexual dysfunction	7. bupropion, nefazodone, citalopram

[1]*Note:* Many antidepressants are quite toxic when taken in overdose. Extreme caution should be exercised in prescribing to high-risk suicidal patients.

[2]Weight gain is rare in the acute phase of treatment with SSRIs, however with prolonged use approximately 10% of patients will experience noticeable weight gain.

recurrence).* Continued (lifelong) treatment provides the best outcome for such individuals. The following guidelines are offered:

1. *First Episode:* at the end of the continuation phase, gradually reduce the dose (over a period of 2–4 weeks) and, assuming no return of depressive symptoms, discontinue. Educate the patient to be alert to any signs of recurrence (e.g., poor sleep, fatigue, etc.) and should this occur, contact the treating doctor as soon as possible to reinstigate treatment.

2. *Second Episode:*

   a. With *"Risk Factors"* which include: family history of mood disorders, first episode occurring prior to the age of 18, and/or most recent episode has severe symptoms: Recommend life-long medication treatment to prevent recurrence.

   b. Without *"Risk Factors"*: gradually discontinue medications.

3. *Third or later episodes.* Recommend life-long medication treatment.

Note: 50–65% of patients with major depression will experience either chronic or recurrent, episodic depressions.

What to Expect

Neuro-researchers have hypothesized that many of the primary symptoms of clinical depression are caused by a dysregulation of certain neurotransmitters (e.g., norepinephrine, dopamine, and/or serotonin). Antidepressant medications are able to restore normal neuronal functioning in key limbic structures in the brain. It is very important to note, however, that these drugs do not act rapidly. It generally requires 2–4 weeks of treatment for symptoms to begin to improve. This is a crucial point. Many, if not most, depressed patients become easily discouraged if there is no relief in a few days. Such patients often discontinue medications prematurely.

Side Effects

Probably owing to their tremendous feelings of hopelessness and pessimism, depressed patients are especially prone to discontinuing treatment prematurely. This is often the case when they encounter side effects which typically emerge long before the therapeutic effects are realized. Thus, choosing medications that are low in side effects is an important rule of thumb. Fortunately, most newer generation antidepressants have a far better side effect profile than older generation tricyclics. Side effects certainly account for treatment failures, however it should be noted that other factors also contribute to treatment drop-outs (see figure 8). It is likely that many drop-outs are due to the prolonged time before the onset of symptomatic improvement and tremendous pessimism that is a cardinal feature of depression.

Figure 8

Only 20% of patients treated in primary care settings receive adequate treatment (i.e. high enough dose and long enough time taking medication) (Agency for Health Care Policy)

Drop-outs due to side effects
First six weeks of treatment

Placebo	3–7%
Tricyclics	25–30%
New generation antidepressants	9–21%

Side Effect Management Considerations: SSRIs

SSRIs are often prescribed for depression owing to their effectiveness and relatively low incidence of side effects. Recently, two later-onset side effects (generally seen 4–6 months into treatment) have been noted. These side effects are a common reason for patient-initiated discontinuation or poor compliance, and are side effects patients seldom report (thus, it is important for the physician to inquire). The side effects include sexual dysfunction (especially inorgasmia) and/or decreased spontaneity and apathy. This last side effect may be spotted by reports by the patient that "I'm feeling depressed again." However, on closer inspection most depressive symptoms continue to be in remission. Rather, the patient is experiencing either a loss of motivation or a decreased sense of emotional aliveness (sometimes including an inability to cry.)

These side-effects can often be successfully managed by the pharmacologic solutions indicated below:

Figure 9

PROBLEM	TREATMENT OPTION
■ Inorgasmia	■ Reduce SSRI dose, or ■ Add buspirone 10–20 mg, b.i.d., or ■ Add cyproheptadine 4–12 mg., p.r.n.
■ Apathy, decreased spontaneity	■ Reduce SSRI dose, or ■ Add bupropion (start low: e.g., 75 mg. b.i.d. and do not exceed 225 mg. q.d.)

Common Treatment Errors To Avoid

- Under-dosing
- Poor compliance
- Co-morbid substance abuse (if not detected, can result in treatment failure of antidepressants. This is a very common reason for inadequate medication response).
- Using benzodiazepines to treat depression (can increase depressive symptoms and may lead to drug dependence/abuse)
- Premature discontinuation
- Rapid discontinuation

KEY POINTS TO COMMUNICATE TO PATIENTS

In prescribing antidepressant medication, patient education is especially important. Listed below are the key points to communicate to patients starting on antidepressants.

1. Onset of clinical action generally takes 2–4 weeks. It will take this long for you to notice a reduction of symptoms.
2. Symptomatic improvement is usually seen primarily in the physiological symptoms (Figure 4). Many of the other symptoms (e.g., depressed mood, low self-esteem, etc.) may respond only partially to medication treatment. These medications are not "happy pills"; they do not totally erase feelings of sadness or emptiness.
3. The best barometers of early medication response generally include improved sleep, less daytime fatigue, and some improvement in emotional control (e.g., less

frequent crying spells or better frustration tolerance). The physician may need to inquire specifically about these symptoms because many depressed people will say "I'm no better," despite the fact that there is symptomatic improvement.

4. There may be side effects. However, side effects can most often be managed by dosage adjustment or by switching to another medication.

5. Total length of treatment varies considerably for individuals. Typically, it may take 4–8 weeks for the major depressive symptoms to subside. It is very important not to discontinue treatment at this point. The acute relapse rate can be as high as 80%. The general rule of thumb is to continue treatment for a period of 6 months beyond the point of symptomatic improvement and then gradually to reduce the dose. Should symptoms return during this medication-reduction phase of treatment, the dosage should again be increased. Medication should be continued for 4–6 weeks before another trial on lower doses. Occasionally, a person may need to be on long-term chronic medication management.

6. Antidepressants are not addictive.

7. You should not drink alcohol when taking antidepressants. Alcohol can block the effects of the antidepressants (although, in clinical practice, many physicians will allow patients on antidepressants to have an occasional drink, but not in excess of one per day).

8. Never discontinue "cold turkey"; this can result in withdrawal symptoms.

9. Two strategies always improve depression: exercise and a reduction of substances that impair sleep (most common: caffeine and alcohol).

Treatment-Resistant Depressions

Generally it is best to start with a typical antidepressant. It is necessary to treat at adequate doses; most treatment failures are due to inadequate doses. Unless side effects are intolerable or a person is a high risk patient (see *Precautions,* pg. 16), standard practice is to push the dose to the upper level of the therapeutic range until symptomatic improvement is attained. If a patient is on a high dose for a period of 3–4 weeks without symptomatic improvement it is unlikely that improvement will occur. If there is a partial response, then a strategy that is often successful is to augment. The most common forms of augmentation are: SSRI plus bupropion (e.g. 150 mg qd), SSRI plus buspirone, SSRI plus low dose stimulant (e.g. methylphenidate, 5-10 mg.) or antidepressant plus low doses of lithium (e.g. 600-900 mg qd). A fairly large number of non-respondents do benefit from augmentation. Should this fail, then a change in the antidepressant medication is in order.

The next step generally is to switch to another typical antidepressant. The choice is guided by two factors: side effect profiles and neurotransmitter action. There is some evidence to suggest that there exist three basic neurochemicals that may be affected in major depressive disorder: norepinephrine, dopamine and serotonin. The various antidepressant medications have different effects on these three neurochemical systems (see Figure 10). Some are considered to have broad spectrum effects ("shotguns") and others are more selective ("bullets"). If your first unsuccessful drug was serotonergic, then the second choice should be a medication targeting norepinephrine or dopamine.

Figure 10

SELECTIVE ACTION OF ANTIDEPRESSANT MEDICATIONS

GENERIC	BRAND	NOREPINEPHRINE	SEROTONIN	MONOAMINE OXIDASE	DOPAMINE
imipramine	Tofranil	+ +	+ + +	0	0
desipramine	Norpramin	+ + + + +	0	0	0
amitriptyline	Elavil	+	+ + + +	0	0
nortriptyline	Aventyl, Pamelor	+ + +	+ +	0	0
protriptyline	Vivactil[1]	+ + + +	+	0	0
trimipramine	Surmontil[1]	+ +	+ +	0	0
doxepin	Sinequan, Adapin[1]	+ + +	+ +	0	0
maprotiline	Ludiomil	+ + + + +	0	0	0
amoxapine	Asendin	+ + + +	+	0	0
venlafaxine	Effexor	+ +	+ + +	0	+
trazodone	Desyrel	0	+ + + + +	0	0
fluoxetine	Prozac	0	+ + + + +	0	0
paroxetine	Paxil	+	+ + + + +	0	0
sertraline	Zoloft	0	+ + + + +	0	0
bupropion	Wellbutrin[2]	+ + +	0	0	+ +
nefazodone	Serzone	+	+ + + +	0	0
fluvoxamine	Luvox	0	+ + + + +	0	0
mirtazapine	Remeron	+ + +	+ + +	0	0
citalopram	Celexa	0	+ + + + +	0	0
escitalopram	Lexapro	0	+ + + + +	0	0
reboxetine	Vestra	+ + + + +	0	0	0
phenelzine	Nardil[3]	+ + +	+ + +	+ + + + +	+ + +
tranylcypromine	Parnate[3]	+ + +	+ + +	+ + + + +	+ + +
isocarboxazid	Marplan[3]	+ + +	+ + +	+ + + + +	+ + +

[1]Uncertain, but likely effects.
[2]Atypical antidepressant. Uncertain effects.
[3]MAOIs increase NE, 5-HT, and DA

What if this fails too? A fourth strategy is to switch to mirtazanine, venlafaxine, or to an MAO inhibitor. Treatment is described below. The final option is electrocovulsive therapy (ECT) which is a highly effective, albeit costly, form of treatment for depression.

Note that the clinician must wait 2 weeks after discontinuing typical antidepressants before beginning an MAOI, and six weeks after discontinuing fluoxetine before a switch to an MAOI. Failure to do so may result in very serious, life-threatening drug interactions.

Dysthymia

Dysthmia is a type of mild, chronic depressive disorder characterized by the following symptoms (which are present almost every day over a period of 2+ years):

- Daytime fatigue
- Negative, pessimistic thinking
- Low self-esteem
- Low motivation, loss of enthusiasm
- Decreased capacity for joy

Evidence from a number of recent studies suggests that 50–55% of patients with dysthymia can respond favorably to a trial on anti-depressant medications. MAOIs and SSRIs appear to be more effective than tricyclics in treating dysthymia (Klein, 1995).

Seasonal Affective Disorder (S.A.D.)

Decreased exposure to photic stimulation has been strongly implicated in cases of S.A.D. This is often a factor in people who work at night, live in geographic areas with significant cloud cover and/or pollution, and in northern climes (Northern hemisphere) during winter months. A full discussion of S.A.D. is beyond the scope of this book, but physicians should be aware of this common clinical condition. Treatment for S.A.D. includes antidepressants (current hypotheses suggest that S.A.D. may be closely tied to serotinergic dysfunction and thus, SSRIs may be medications of choice). Additionally, increased bright light exposure has been shown to be effective (either by use of commercially available light boxes or by encouraging patients to spend a minimum of one hour per day outside . . . of course, without sunglasses).

For a detailed discussion of S.A.D., please see *Winter Blues* by N.E. Rosenthal, Guilford Press, N.Y. (1993).

Pre-menstrual Dysphoric Disorder (PMDD)

Approximately 5% of women experience severe mood changes premenstrually. This disorder is characterized by the tremendous regularity of mood symptoms (depression, irritability or anxiety) seen for a few days prior to ovulation. Serotinergic dysregulation has been implicated and treatment with SSRIs is often a successful strategy. Currently, there is some debate whether or not it is necessary to treat PMDD continuously (i.e., all month-long) or on a P.R.N. basis. All other types of depression require chronic treatment, however, some women with PMDD *may* respond to P.R.N. dosing only during the symptomatic time of the month.

Psychotic Depressions

Psychotic symptoms may be seen in cases of unipolar depression and bipolar disorder, and occur also in the context of postpartum and menopausal depressions. They usually manifest with severe vegetative symptoms, delusions (especially somatic delusions, extreme beliefs regarding worthlessness, and paranoid thinking) and occasionally, auditory hallucinations.

Antidepressants alone or antipsychotics alone are generally ineffective. Almost always the treatment of choice includes a combination of antidepressants and antipsychotics. Electroconvulsive therapy (E.C.T.) may be both necessary and effective in more severe cases. Finally, please keep in mind that these patients are very high risk for suicide. Referral to a psychiatrist and possibly hospitalization are recommended.

Precautions: Tricyclic Antidepressants

The following patients should either not be treated or treated cautiously with tricyclics: immediate post-MI patients, epileptics, patients with narrow-angle glaucoma, and pregnant women. The physician should consult package inserts and the *Physicians' Desk Reference* for more details regarding precautions and contradictions.

Precautions: Selective Serotonin Reuptake Inhibitors

Drug-drug interactions can sometimes be dangerous. SSRIs should be used *cautiously* with the following medications (Figure 11):

Figure 11

- MAO Inhibitors—never use with SSRIs (very dangerous/fatal)
- Tricyclic antidepressants (may increase TCA levels)
- Lithium (may increase lithium levels)
- Carbamazepine (may increase carbamazepine levels)
- St. John's Wort (may be dangerous)

Note: this list is not exhaustive, but includes common drug-drug interactions

Precautions: Watch for Bipolar Disorder

Patients with a personal or family history of bipolar disorder often present with depressive symptoms. They may or may not reveal a history of mania. Caution should be exercised in prescribing since all antidepressants can precipitate a rapid shift from depression into mania. It is always advisable to ask the patient (and family members) if there has been a family history of bipolar illness or if any of the following have been present for more than one or two days:

- Decreased need for sleep, but without daytime fatigue
- Rapid, pressured speech
- High levels of energy
- Racing thoughts

If a patient reports any of these symptoms, they should be considered bipolar until proven otherwise. Treatment should include co-administration of an antidepressant and a mood stabilizer (see Chapter 3).

MAO Inhibitors

Three commonly used MAOIs, phenelzine, isocarboxazid, and tranylcypromine have been shown to be as effective as tricyclics in a number of studies. However, shortly after their introduction into the United States in the 1950s there were reports of severe reactions in some patients, which resulted in great concern in the medical community. The drugs interact with certain medications (sympathomimetic amines) and with certain foods (containing tyramine, a natural byproduct of bacterial fermentation processes, found in many cheeses, some wines and beers, and foods such as chopped liver, broad beans, chocolate, snails, etc.). (See Appendix B.) The interaction resulted in a severe hypertensive crisis, which for a number of patients was fatal. So for many years these medications were abandoned because doctors viewed them as unsafe. However, especially in Europe, doctors recognized that these drugs had clinical utility and could be safely used if certain dietary restrictions were followed.

MAOIs should be considered as a third or fourth line treatment choice, should other antidepressants fail. Additionally, some studies indicate that MAOIs may be the drug of choice for some types of affective disorders including atypical depressions presenting primarily with anxiety and phobic symptoms, masked depression (e.g., hypochondriasis), and dysthymia.

Otherwise, guidelines for treatment and clinical response are similar to those previously described for typical antidepressants. The one exception is the important dietary/medication restrictions that must be observed (see Appendix B, patient handout for specific restrictions).

Notes on Over-the-Counter Products

Two OTC products have some research support for treatment of depression: St. John's Wort (SJW) and SAM-e. Both appear to have favorable side effect profiles and efficacy. SJW has been shown to have a significant impact on hepatic metabolism and may result in numerous drug-drug interactions (some of which have resulted in fatalities). Please check with a pharmacist regarding the latest findings regarding such interactions. Additionally, when switching from SJW to a prescription antidepressant, the wash out period is five days. Combining SJW and antidepressants can be dangerous. Studies are now in progress at NIMH and final conclusions regarding efficacy and safety should await the outcome of these investigations.

Books to Recommend to Patients

1. Preston, J. (2000). *You Can Beat Depression: A Guide to Prevention and Recovery* (second edition), Impact Publishers, Atascadero, CA.
2. Jefferson, J. and Greist, J.H. (1999). *Depression and Antidepressants: A Guide,* Madison Institute of Medicine, Madison, Wisconsin.
3. Preston, J. (2001). *Lift Your Mood Now: Simple Exercises for Beating the Blues.* New Harbinger Publications, Oakland.

Chapter 3   Bipolar Illness

DIAGNOSIS

Major Clinical Features and Differential Diagnosis

The diagnosis of a bipolar disorder is based in two sources of data: the current clinical picture (depression or mania) and a clear history of both manic and depressive episodes. The depressive episodes may range from minor to major depressive syndromes as outlined in Chapter 2. Manic episodes typically are described as either full blown or less intense manic episodes, referred to as hypomania.

It is important to rule out medical causes of bipolar illness. (See Figures 1 and 2 in Chapter 2 and Figures 12 and 13.)

Figure 12

COMMON DISORDERS THAT MAY CAUSE MANIA

- Brain tumors
- CNS syphilis
- Delirium (due to various causes)
- Encephalitis
- Influenza
- Metabolic changes associated with hemodialysis
- Metastatic squamous adenocarcinoma
- Multiple sclerosis
- Q fever

Figure 13

DRUGS THAT MAY CAUSE MANIA

- amphetamines
- bromides
- cocaine
- antidepressants
- isoniazid
- procarbazine
- steroids

Several classification schemes for bipolar disorders have been proposed by various authors. The three most clinically useful classifications are outlined below:

A. BIPOLAR I vs. BIPOLAR II

1. *Bipolar I* This disorder fits the more classic description of bipolar illness with clearly recognized episodes of depression and mania.

2. *Bipolar II* This disorder presents with obvious episodes of depression; but the manic phases of the illness are often less intense, unrecognized, and thus not reported by the patient. If you inquire about manic episodes, the patient will give the impression that none have occurred. The best ways to diagnose such conditions are either to witness a hypomanic episode clinically or to carefully inquire about the history. In particular, if hypomanic episodes are suspected, the most important question to ask is, "Have you ever had a period of time when you didn't need as much sleep?" A decreased need for sleep and a lack of daytime fatigue are red flags for hypomania.

B. TYPICAL BIPOLAR vs. RAPID CYCLING BIPOLAR DISORDERS

In the more typical bipolar patient, depressive and manic episodes last for several weeks to several months, often with periods of normal mood occurring between periods of depression and mania. When there are two or more episodes of *both* depression and mania, (e.g., depression-mania-depression-mania) within a year, this is referred to as "rapid cycling." Sometimes rapid cyclers can dramatically switch moods from week to week or even day to day.

C. DYSPHORIC MANIA (or MIXED MANIA)

This is a diagnostic term which describes patients that have concurrent manic and depressive symptoms (e.g., increased activity or agitation, pressured speech, suicidal ideas, and feelings of worthlessness).

The subclassifications of Bipolar I and Bipolar II, typical vs. rapid cycling, and dysphoric mania are important because they have different treatment implications.

Target Symptoms

The target symptoms vary depending on the current phase of the illness. Major depressive symptoms are listed in Chapter 2 (Figures 3 and 4). Manic episodes are identified by the following clinical features (see Figure 14).

MEDICATIONS USED TO TREAT BIPOLAR ILLNESS

When Do You Prescribe Medications?

Treatment of bipolar disorders has two goals. The first goal is the reduction of current symptoms, and the second is the prevention of relapse. Bipolar disorders

Figure 14

SYMPTOMS OF MANIA[1]

■ A pronounced and persistent mood of euphoria (elevated or expansive mood) or irritability and at least three of the following:

■ Grandiosity or elevated self-esteem

■ Decreased need for sleep

■ Rapid, pressured speech (Often these people are hard, if not impossible, to interrupt.)

■ Racing thoughts

■ Distractibility

■ Increased activity or psychomotor agitation

■ Behavior that reflects expansiveness (lacking restraint in emotional expression) and poor judgment, such as increased sexual promiscuity, gambling, buying sprees, giving away money, etc.

----

[1]Adapted from APA, 1987 (with permission), p. 217. Also see Questions 13–16 on the History and Personal Data Questionnaire (Appendix A.).

are invariably recurring and thus prophylactic treatment is warranted. Strong evidence indicates that failure to continue treatment can and often leads not only to relapse, but to a progressively worsening condition. Subsequent episodes tend to become more and more severe and can, at times, become treatment refractory.

Choosing Medication

The primary medication used to treat this disorder is lithium. However a number of other drugs have been found to be effective as adjuncts or alternatives to lithium. We will describe standard treatment with lithium and then comment on the role of other medications.

Lithium has two primary effects: It stabilizes mood, and in many instances it can prevent relapse (or at least lessen the intensity of subsequent episodes) if treatment is on an ongoing basis. Lithium seems to be somewhat more effective in preventing relapse of mania rather than depression.

Prescribing Treatment

The treatment of bipolar disorders can be quite complex. Generally a referral to a specialist is recommended.

If the presenting phase is a manic episode. Often, especially if the patient is quite agitated, out of control or psychotic, the initial plan is to begin treatment with *both* a mood stabilizer and an antipsychotic medication (e.g. olanzapine). The antipsychotics seem to improve behavioral control more rapidly. With most mood stabilizers, the patient may require 10 days to show a clinical response. Once mood has been stabilized, the antipsychotic may be phased out. Alternatively, high potency benzodiazepines can be used in place of antipsychotics (e.g., clonazepam).

Treatment with lithium is initiated after necessary lab tests are conducted (see Figure 16.) Generally the starting dose is 600 or 900 mg./day given in divided doses. The therapeutic range and toxic range of lithium are very close to one another. Thus it is necessary to gradually increase the dose while carefully monitoring blood levels. Most patients must reach a level between 1.0 and 1.2 mEq/L. Not infrequently the level may need to be higher to obtain symptomatic improvement (1.2 to 1.6), but on these higher levels, side effects are more common and compliance is poorer. On occasion, patients may need and tolerate blood levels up to 2.0 mEq/L. However, there is increased risk of toxicity at such doses. Generally, daily doses range from 1200-3000 mg. Once mood is adequately stabilized, the dose can be lowered somewhat (0.8-1.0 mEq/L) for maintenance treatment.

If the presenting phase is a depressive episode. Antidepressants alone in the treatment of bipolar depression can cause significant problems, by provoking a rapid shift into mania (and also may increase the subsequent frequency of episodes; i.e.

Figure 15

DECISION TREE FOR TREATMENT OF BIPOLAR DISORDERS

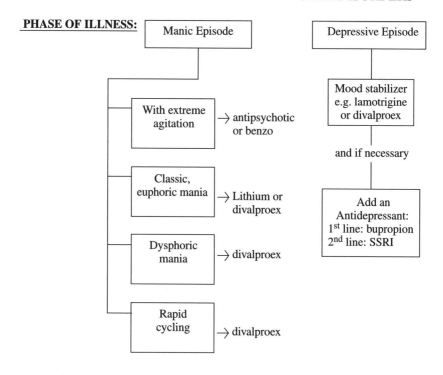

causing cycle acceleration). Thus, typically the treatment of choice is to use a mood stabilizer (however, note that only two mood stabilizers have been found to have antidepressant properties: lamotrigine and divalproex). Should this strategy fail, an antidepressant may be added to the mood stabilizer. Bipolar depression is especially difficult to treat and in most instances, a referral to a psychiatrist is in order.

Side Effects of Lithium and Signs of Toxicity

Major side effects include nausea, diarrhea, vomiting, fine hand tremor, sedation, muscular weakness, polyuria, polydypsia, edema, weight gain and a dry mouth. Adverse effects from chronic use may include leukocytosis (reversible upon discontinuation of lithium), hypothyroidism and goiter, acne, psoriasis, teratogenesis (first trimester, although the risk is low), nephrogenic diabetes insipidus (reversible), and kidney damage.

Signs of toxicity include lethargy, ataxia, slurred speech, tinnitus, severe nausea/vomiting, tremor, arrhythmias, hypotension, seizures, shock, delirium, coma, and even death. Since the toxic range is near to the therapeutic range, blood levels and adverse effects must be monitored closely. In addition, a number of other clinical lab tests should be conducted at the beginning of treatment and periodically thereafter (see Figure 16).

Figure 16

CLINICAL LAB TESTS FOR PATIENTS TAKING LITHIUM

- NA (Sodium)
- Ca (Calcium)
- P (Phosphorus)
- EKG
- Creatinine
- Urinalysis
- Complete CBC
- Thyroid battery (with TSH)

Listed below are the key points that should be communicated to patients starting treatment with lithium.

KEY POINTS TO COMMUNICATE TO PATIENTS

1. Lithium is a medication that treats your current emotional problem and will also be helpful in preventing relapse. So it will be important to continue with treatment after the current episode is resolved.

2. Since the therapeutic and toxic dosage ranges are so close, we must monitor your blood level closely. This will be done more frequently at first and every several months thereafter. Never increase your dose without first consulting with your physician.

3. Lithium and other mood stabilizers are not addictive.

4. Many side effects can be reduced/minimized by taking divided doses or may subside as treatment progresses.

5. Bipolar disorders often run in families. Any relatives that have pronounced mood swings should be alerted to the possibility of a treatable condition and the need for professional evaluation. (The yield on this maneuver is high, since medical awareness of bipolar disorder is still low, especially with milder forms, and family history is impressively often positive for this disorder.)

6. You and your family need to be aware that this is a biological disorder, not a moral defect or a character flaw. When severe, you may not always be able to control your behavior, necessitating that practical steps be taken to protect all concerned from poor judgment during episodes.

7. Many self-help groups have been developed to provide support for bipolar patients and their families. In this community, the local self-help group is ____, and you can find out more information by calling ____.

Common Treatment Errors to Avoid

- Lithium: very toxic thus warrants close monitoring (especially in suicidal patients. Note: suicides occur frequently not only in depressed but also manic patients)
- Poor compliance
- Discontinuation: note: bipolar patients need life-long treatment to avoid relapse. Patient or physician-initiated discontinuation can and does result in frequent relapses. And, subsequent episodes often are more severe and may become treatment-resistant. If discontinuation must occur, it is strongly recommended that it be done gradually (e.g. over a period of 6 weeks).

Specialized Treatments for Subtypes of Bipolar Disorder

In addition to standard lithium treatment, many researchers and clinicians have suggested treatment options for certain bipolar subtypes (see Figure 17).

Figure 17

SPECIALIZED TREATMENTS FOR SUBTYPES OF BIPOLAR DISORDERS

SUBTYPE	MEDICATION ALTERNATIVES
Bipolar II	Lamotrigine or divalproex
Rapid Cyclers	Divalproex or carbamazepine
Dysphoric Mania	Divalproex

Newer Treatment Alternatives

For treatment refractory patients, the following medications can be used (as sole agents or to augment standard treatments): anticonvulsants: Lamictal (lamotrigine), Neurontin (gabapentin),Topamax (topiramate), Trileptal (oxcarbazepine) (note, the use of these anticonvulsants for bipolar disorder, although common, is off label), atypical antipsychotics (e.g. olanzapine) or Klonopin (clonazepam) for mania; high doses of T_3 (e.g. 150-200 micrograms) for rapid cycling; the calcium channel blocker verapamil. In clinical practice, only 33% of patients remain on monotherapy; i.e. combination/augmentation is frequently required (e.g. lithium and divalproex).

For details on newer treatment approaches see the following:

Practice Guidelines for Treatment of Patients with Bi-Polar Disorder.

Supplement to the *American Journal of Psychiatry,* December, 1994: American Psychiatric Press: 1-800-368-5777.

Books to Recommend to Patients

1. Jamison, K. R. (1997). *Unquiet Mind,* Random House, New York.

2. Mondimore, F. (1999). *Bipolar Disorder: A Guide for Patients and Families,* Johns Hopkins University Press.

3. Papolos, D. and Papolos, J. (1999). *The Bipolar Child.* Broadway Books, New York.

Chapter 4   Anxiety Disorders

DIAGNOSIS

Major Clinical Features and Differential Diagnosis

Six different anxiety disorders are seen in clinical practice. An accurate diagnosis is important as the treatments vary. There is no one treatment appropriate for all anxiety disorders. It is important to distinguish between the following: (1) generalized anxiety disorder (G.A.D.), (2) stress related anxiety, (3) panic disorder, (4) social phobias, (5) medical illnesses presenting with anxiety symptoms, and (6) anxiety symptoms as a part of a primary mental disorder (e.g., depression, schizophrenia).

Before outlining the main features of each disorder, it is necessary to define two terms: panic attacks and anxiety symptoms. Panic attacks are very brief but extremely intense surges of anxiety. The major differences between a panic attack and more generalized anxiety symptoms are differences in the onset, duration, and intensity. Panic attacks often "come out of the blue" (i.e., not necessarily provoked by stress), they come on suddenly (the full attack reaching its peak in from one-to-ten minutes), are *extremely* intense, last from 1–30 minutes, and then subside. The patient feels as if he will actually die or go crazy. We are not talking about uneasiness; we are talking about full-blown panic. The person may continue to feel nervous or upset for several hours, but the attack itself lasts only a matter of minutes. If a patient says, "I've had a continuous panic attack for the past three days," he may be having intense anxiety symptoms, but not a true panic attack. In other anxiety disorders, anxiety symptoms can be very unpleasant, but are much less intense; they also can be prolonged or generalized (i.e., present most of the day and last from days to years). The distinction between "symptoms" and "attacks" is very important when it comes to treatment. Please refer to Figure 18.

The six anxiety syndromes can be distinguished by the following characteristics:

1. *Generalized Anxiety Disorder.* The key here is *long-term,* low level, fairly continuous anxiety. Patients with this disorder *may* have no specific current life stressors. To them, daily living provokes anxiety. Such people are chronic

---

Note: Obsessive-Compulsive disorder and Post-traumatic stress disorder are discussed in Chapter 6.

Figure 18

SYMPTOMS OF ANXIETY[1]

- Trembling, feeling shaky, restlessness, muscle tension
- Shortness of breath, smothering sensation
- Tachycardia (rapid heartbeat)
- Sweating and cold hands and feet
- Lightheadedness and dizziness
- Paresthesias (tingling of the skin)
- Diarrhea and/or frequent urination
- Feelings of unreality (derealization)
- Initial insomnia (difficulty falling asleep)
- Impaired attention and concentration
- Nervousness, edginess, or tension

---

[1]Adapted from APA, 1987 (with permission), p. 253.

worriers, always 'what-if-ing" (e.g., "What if I get fired?" "What if my check bounces?" "What if my wife leaves me?").

2. *Stress-related Anxiety.* The patient with this disorder typically functions well. However, the anxiety symptoms have recently emerged in the face of major life stresses (e.g., a serious family illness, a marital separation, etc.).

3. *Panic Disorder.* This is characterized by repeated episodes of full-blown panic, as described in the discussion of panic attacks. Often phobias will also develop.

4. *Social Phobias.* Anxiety is experienced only when the person is in social/interpersonal settings, e.g., public speaking, asking someone out for a date, social gatherings.

5. *Medical Illnesses, and Medications Presenting with Anxiety Symptoms.* Certain diseases/conditions can at times result in biochemical changes that produce anxiety symptoms. If someone complains of nervousness or anxiety, it should never be assumed that it is simply an emotional disorder until medical causes have been ruled out (Figure 19). Likewise, a number of medications and over-the-counter products can cause pronounced anxiety symptoms (Figure 20).

6. *Anxiety as a Part of a Primary Mental Disorder.* Anxiety frequently accompanies many mental disorders (e.g., depression, schizophrenia, organic brain syndromes, substance abuse).

Figure 19

COMMON DISORDERS THAT MAY CAUSE ANXIETY

- Adrenal tumor
- Alcoholism
- Angina pectoris
- Cardiac arrhythmia
- CNS degenerative diseases
- Cushing's disease
- Coronary insufficiency
- Delirium[1]

- Hypoglycemia
- Hyperthyroidism
- Meniere's disease (early stages)
- Mitral valve prolapse[2]
- Parathyroid disease
- Partial-complex seizures
- Post-concussion syndrome
- Premenstrual syndrome

[1]Delirium can occur as a result of many toxic/metabolic conditions and often produces anxiety and agitation.

[2]The mitral valve prolapse probably does not cause anxiety, but it has been found that MVP and anxiety disorders often coexist. This may be due to some underlying common genetic factor.

Figure 20

DRUGS THAT MAY CAUSE ANXIETY

- Amphetamines
- Appetite suppressants
- Asthma medications
- Caffeine
- CNS depressants (withdrawal)
- Cocaine
- Nasal decongestants
- Steroids

ANTIANXIETY MEDICATION* TREATMENT

When Do You Prescribe Antianxiety Medications?

Treatment differs depending on the diagnosis, so each disorder will be addressed separately.

1. *Generalized Anxiety Disorder (G.A.D.).* Many physicians have tried to treat this disorder with benzodiazepines. This presents two problems: (1) In the long

*Also referred to as minor tranquilizers, anxiolytics, and benzodiazepines. These terms will be used interchangeably.

run, such treatment is often not very effective. (2) Patients can develop tolerance/dependence problems with chronic benzodiazepine use. Many clinicians think that G.A.D. is primarily a psychological (not biological) disorder and recommend psychotherapy. However, SSRIs, venlafaxine and buspirone hydrochloride, have been shown to be effective in treating G.A.D. An added feature of these medications is that patients do not develop dependence or tolerance.

2. *Stress-related anxiety.* Minor tranquilizers are very helpful in reducing anxiety symptoms (especially insomnia and restlessness) which accompany acute situational stress. The most important issue to consider is whether or not the stress is acute and likely to be of short duration. Antianxiety medications should only be used for a period of 1–4 weeks. If it is clear that this is just one in a series of chronic life crises, it is probably best not to prescribe benzodiazepines. (see below)

3. *Panic disorder.* One isolated panic attack is generally insufficient evidence of true panic disorder. However, four or more true attacks within a period of one month suggest panic disorder. Look for spontaneous attacks (most "come out of the blue") episodes that last a matter of minutes (not hours or days). Many patients with other types of disorders say they have panic attacks but on close inspection, many do not.

4. *Social phobias.* Generally, social phobias are not treated medically but with psychotherapy and behavioral approaches. In some cases beta blockers, MAO inhibitors, venlafaxine or SSRIs have been helpful.

5. *Medical illnesses/medications causing anxiety symptoms.* In almost all instances, the treatment of choice is to treat the primary medical illness or to discontinue the offending drug. Be cautious in stopping certain drugs; for instance, if a patient stops drinking coffee abruptly, he may have significant withdrawal symptoms which mimic anxiety. Such drugs must be gradually withdrawn.

6. *Anxiety symptoms as a part of another primary mental disorder.* Treat the primary disorder. Minor tranquilizers are usually not indicated.

Choosing a Medication

Antianxiety medications fall into five groups (see Figure 21). The primary choice of medication is based on the diagnosis. Secondarily, one should consider certain problematic side effects such as sedation and rapidity of absorption (rapid absorption may be associated with a euphoric "rush").

Prescribing Treatment

1. *Generalized Anxiety Disorder.* There are several options, including buspirone. Unlike the benzodiazepines, buspirone is slow acting. It often requires 2–6 weeks

of treatment before symptomatic improvement. The major problem encountered with this medication is premature discontinuation by the patient. Patients often expect quick results from medications. It is important to educate the patient about onset of action. Buspirone can be effective in treating many symptoms of G.A.D., but it does not seem to decrease panic attacks. Buspirone must be taken every day; it is not a medication that is taken only when the patient feels anxious. SSRIs or venlafaxine may also be beneficial in treating G.A.D. If patients fail to respond to buspirone, venlafaxine, or SSRIs, if symptoms are severe, and if there is no history of alcohol or other substance abuse, benzodiazepines can be used to treat G.A.D.

2. *Stress-Related Anxiety.* All benzodiazepines are effective in treating acute stress-induced anxiety. (See Figure 21). The most important considerations in choosing a medication have to do with side effects and medication half life. The most common side effect is sedation. Intense restlessness or agitation may require a more sedating drug; however, in most instances it is better to use low sedation benzodiazepines to reduce daytime anxiety. Of course many anxious patients will present with a sleep disturbance. Insomnia will be addressed below. A second side effect is the so-called euphoric "rush" secondary to the peak in blood level of medication. Such a peak creates a good deal of sedation and can be useful if the goal is to induce sleep, but the euphoric experience can lead to abuse. In addiction-prone individuals it is best to choose a drug that avoids or minimizes this effect. Finally the half life of a medication is an important variable when it comes to discontinuing the drug. Those medications listed that have a shorter half life may need to be discontinued *very* gradually so as to avoid withdrawal symptoms.

Dosage ranges vary widely as seen in Figure 21. However, a typical starting dose of lorazepam, for instance, is 0.5 mg. b.i.d. or t.i.d. Such a dose should be increased every three days as needed until a final range of 2–6 mg./day is achieved. The goal is to provide some symptomatic relief over a period of from 1–4 weeks. Should a person still experience significant anxiety after this period of time, a reassessment of the diagnosis is in order.

It has long been held that long term use of benzodiazepines is contraindicated. Although this is often true, it is not always the case. Investigations into chronic benzodiazepine use have shed new light on this clinical practice. Uhlenhuth, et al. (1988, p. 161) report that " . . . many patients continue to derive benefit from long-term treatment with benzodiazepines; and . . . attitudes strongly against the use of these drugs may be depriving many anxious patients of appropriate treatment." The key is to monitor closely for signs of increasing dosage, especially as the patient may be increasing dosage without medical advice. If in doubt, don't hesitate to get a blood level and to share your concerns openly with the patient. Addiction to benzodiazepines that arise in the course of the treatment of anxiety should be treated for what it is: an occasional and serious side effect. *Always* discontinue benzodiazepines gradually (e.g., if the patient takes 1.5 mg. of alprazolam, q.d., then each week the daily dose should

Figure 21

ANTIANXIETY MEDICATIONS

Disorder	Medication Generic	Brand	Usual Daily Dosage Range	Rapidity of Absorption	½ Life (Hours)
1. G.A.D.	buspirone	BuSpar	5–40 mg.	+	2–8
	SSRIs[1]				
2. Stress-Related Anxiety	diazepam	Valium	5–40 mg.	+++++	20–50
	chlordiazepoxide	Librium	15–100 mg.	+++	5–30
	oxazepam	Serax	30–120 mg.	++	5–20
	clorazepate	Tranxene	15–60 mg.	++++	30–100
	lorazepam	Ativan	2–6 mg.	+++	10–15
	prazepam	Centrax	20–60 mg.	+	30–100
	alprazolam	Xanax	.25–4 mg.	+++	6–20
	clonazepam	Klonopin	.5–4 mg.	+	80
3. Panic Disorder	alprazolam	Xanax	.25–.8 mg.	+++	6–20
	lorazepam	Ativan	2–6 mg.	+++	10–15
	clonazepam	Klonopin	.5–4 mg.	+	80
	antidepressants[1]				
	MAO Inhibitors[1]				
4. Social Phobia	propranolol	Inderal	20–80mg.		
	SSRIs[1]				
	venlafaxine[1]				
	MAO Inhibitors[1]				
5. Stress-Related Initial Insomnia[2]	flurazepam	Dalmane	15–30 mg.	+++++	40–250[3]
	temazepam	Restoril	15–30 mg.	+++++	10–20
	triazolam	Halcion	.25–.5 mg.	+++++	2–3
	quazepam	Doral	7.5–15 mg.	+++++	39
	zolpidem	Ambien	5–10 mg.	++++	2–3
	estazolam	Prosom	2–4 mg.	+++++	10–24
	zaleplon	Sonata	5–10 mg.	+++++	1–2

[1]See Chapter 2, Figure 5.
[2]Initial insomnia: difficulty falling asleep.
[3]Active metabolite (norflurazepam)

be reduced by 0.25 mg. This slow taper is especially important with short half-life benzodiazepines).

3. *Stress-Induced Insomnia.* Benzodiazepine sedative-hypnotics can be a safe and effective treatment for transient initial insomnia. (Recall that middle insomnia and early morning awakening are more indicative of depression and therefore should not be treated with benzodiazepines). Again, in most cases treatment is initiated only if the insomnia is precipitated by recent environmental stress and is not a chronic problem. Chronic insomnia is extremely hard

to treat. Note that the newer drug zolpidem tartrate is not a benzodiazepine and studies to-date show that dependence is less likely with this medication. For this reason, it may be a safe alternative in individuals with a substance abuse history. Typical dosages for the various sedatives are listed in Figure 21. Another popular drug of choice that has no addiction potential is the sedating antidepressant trazodone (dosing: 25–100 mg. qhs).

4. *Panic Disorder.* The treatment of panic disorder has two discrete phases.

   Phase One: Eliminate or reduce the frequency or intensity of the panic attacks with antipanic drugs. There are three main groups of antipanic drugs. Let's discuss the pros and cons of each.

   a. High potency benzodiazepines and like compounds (e.g., alprazolam, lorazepam, and clonazepam)

      Pros. Very effective. It works quickly. It also reduces anticipatory anxiety.

      Cons. Although some patients respond to low doses (0.25 mg t.i.d.), most require much larger doses (3–8 mg/day for alprazolam, 2–4 mg/day for clonazepam), and at these higher doses, sedation is a very common problem. With prolonged use, tolerance can develop. *Very* gradual discontinuation is required to avoid withdrawal symptoms.

   b. Antidepressants: tricyclics, selective serotonin re-uptake inhibitors (SSRIs), venlafaxine, mirtazapine.

      Pros. Effective in reducing attacks. Can treat concurrent depression. Can be used for prolonged periods of time without risk of tolerance/dependence.

      Cons. Side effects (see Chapter 2) and delayed onset of action (2–4 weeks before symptomatic improvement). Treat in the same way and same dosage levels as you would use to treat depression. Some patients experience an initial increase in panic attacks; these are usually managed well with short term use of a benzodiazepine, as necessary. (Note: bupropion is one antidepressant that apparently is not effective in treating panic attacks).

   c. MAO Inhibitors

      Pros. Very effective. Can treat concurrent depression. Can be used for prolonged periods of time without risk of tolerance/dependence.

      Cons. Delayed onset of action (2–4 weeks) and medication/dietary restrictions as outlined in Chapter 2. As with typical antidepressants, treat as you would treat depression.

   Phase Two. Patients not only have the attacks, but develop significant anticipatory anxiety, phobias, and avoidance (a strong urge to avoid situations in which they have experienced prior panic attacks, e.g., to avoid crowded stores or driving on freeways). These problems frequently do not spontaneously remit when the panic attacks are eliminated. People continue to have intense worries that "It could happen again." Phase two involves gradual reexposure to feared situations. So, for instance, if a person is afraid of having an attack at the grocery store, he must gradually approach the feared situation. Only by repeated exposure to the situation and by a series of experiences without panic will the patient's anticipatory anxiety and avoidance diminish. The keys to successful graded reexposure are (1) to first effectively control or reduce attacks with medication and then (2) to have the patient very gradually face the phobic situation. To be effective, exposures should last from 60–90 minutes.

The duration of the underlying biochemical dysfunction is quite variable. Some people may be treated medically for six months and gradually withdrawn from medication. Others may need years of continued treatment. (Most patients are treated for 18–24 months.) Like depression, the strategy with any of the antipanic drugs is to achieve symptomatic relief and then continue to treat for at least 6 months. At that point, a medication-reduction trial may be initiated. If necessary, treatment can be resumed if panic symptoms reemerge.

5. Social Phobias. In most cases psychotherapy is the treatment of choice. Psychotropic medications have been used, however, in two types of social phobia. Some social phobics are extremely sensitive to rejection and this is why they are fearful of social interactions. Clinical data indicate that these patients may benefit from MAO inhibitors, venlafaxine, or SSRIs. A second type of phobia, stage fright/public speaking phobia, has been successfully treated by beta blockers such as propanolol (usually 20–40 mg., 1 hour prior to performing). Beta blockers do not eliminate the centrally mediated, subjective sense of anxiety, but do quite effectively reduce many peripheral somatic symptoms of anxiety, e.g., tachycardia, trembling.

Common Treatment Errors to Avoid

- Prescribing benzodiazepines to a patient with a personal or family history of substance abuse (high risk of abusing the benzodiazepine). Watch for patient requests for higher and higher doses.
- "Cold turkey" discontinuation or rapid taper of benzodiazepines (can result in significant withdrawal symptoms. 1–3 month gradual taper advised).
- Misdiagnosis: failure to recognize depression or an emerging psychotic illness and treating with benzodiazepines (can worsen depression and fail to treat psychosis).
- Over sedation with benzodiazepines in the treatment of day-time anxiety.
- Benzodiazepines in treating elderly patients can cause cognitive impairment and contribute to unsteady gait and falls. Use with caution.

IN EVERY CASE, REMEMBER

Some degree of stress and anxiety is a common part of normal, daily living. Medication treatment should only be initiated if symptoms are significantly intense and severely interfere with normal functioning.

When you prescribe any kind of medication to control anxiety, it is essential to discuss the following key points with the patient:

KEY POINTS TO COMMUNICATE TO PATIENTS

Generalized Anxiety Disorder
1. If buspirone, venlafaxine, or SSRIs are prescribed, you should expect that it will take from 2–6 weeks to notice symptomatic improvement. Daily doses are required. This is not a medication that you take only as needed.
2. Often medication treatment is not enough and psychotherapy, stress management, relaxation training, and biofeedback are helpful adjuncts to medical treatment.

Stress-Related Anxiety
1. The following analogy is helpful. Pain killers can reduce suffering when you have a toothache, but at some point you must fix or pull the tooth. Likewise, minor tranquilizers do not cure people, but they temporarily reduce suffering. You must do something to alter the basic source of stress if lasting recovery is to be achieved. Minor tranquilizers are only for short-term use.
2. Do not abruptly discontinue minor tranquilizers, especially if they have been taken daily for several weeks. Cold-turkey discontinuation can result in withdrawal syndromes (many withdrawal symptoms are almost identical to symptoms of anxiety).
3. Do not drink any kind of alcohol if you are taking a minor tranquilizer.

Panic Disorder
1. There is strong evidence that panic disorder is a biochemical dysfunction, not a psychological disorder. It can often be very successfully treated with medications.
2. Medication must be taken each day. The treatment is prophylactic and not a medication that you only take as needed.
3. The medication treats *only* the panic attacks. Once these are adequately controlled, you will need to enter Phase Two of treatment (graded reexposure) to deal with anticipatory anxiety and avoidance. In many cases this is best done with the help of a therapist familiar with behavioral techniques.
4. If MAO inhibitors are used, you must understand the dietary and medication restrictions and sign a consent form.
5. If alprazolam, lorazepam, or clonazepam are used, you must never abruptly discontinue it (medication reduction should be done gradually, generally 0.25 to 0.5 mg. per day per week).
6. If treated by antidepressants or MAOIs, it may take 2–4 weeks before you notice symptomatic changes.

Figure 22

DECISION TREE FOR DIAGNOSIS AND TREATMENT OF ANXIETY

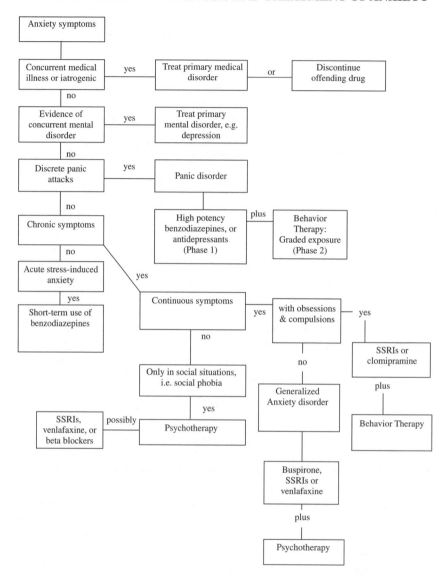

Social Phobias

1. If medication is used (MAOI, SSRI, venlafaxine, or beta blockers), this must be accompanied by exposure (i.e., you must be willing to enter certain social situations and test out the water).
2. Psychotherapy is also indicated.

Books to Recommend to Patients

1. Beckfield, D. (1994). *Master Your Panic,* Impact Publishers, San Luis Obispo, CA.
2. Greist, J. H. and Jefferson, J. (2001). *Panic Disorder and Agoraphobia: A Guide,* Madison Institute of Medicine, Madison, Wisconsin.

Chapter 5   Psychotic Disorders

DIAGNOSIS

Major Clinical Features and Differential Diagnosis

For practical purposes three major psychotic disorders are described: (1) Schizo-phrenia (and schizophrenic-like disorders), (2) psychotic mood disorders, and (3) psychosis associated with neurological conditions.

Before discussing differential diagnosis, let's first briefly define *psychosis*. Psychosis is not an illness; it is a symptom associated with a number of disorders. The hallmark of psychosis is impaired reality testing (impaired ability to perceive reality). The loss of contact with reality can take many forms: severe confusional states, delusions (bizarre, unrealistic thoughts), hallucinations, and marked im-pairment in judgement and reasoning. Having psychotic symptoms does not in itself imply a specific etiology; causes are varied. The three groups of psychotic disorders mentioned above are distinguished by the following characteristics:

1. *Schizophrenia*. Schizophrenia is generally a recurring illness; people diag-nosed as schizophrenic are prone to repeated psychotic episodes. It is helpful to think about three types of schizophrenia:

    a. *Positive Symptom Schizophrenia*. This type of schizophrenia is also re-ferred to as dopaminergic schizophrenia because of its presumed etiology: a hyperactive dopamine system. Positive systems are active, florid delu-sions and hallucinations; agitation and emotional dyscontrol. There are two subtypes:

        1. *Schizophreniform disorder* (Brief psychotic reaction). This disorder looks like schizophrenia but remits quicker and often does not recur.

        2. *Schizophrenia, per se.* This is a recurring or chronic disorder.

    b. *Negative Symptom Schizophrenia*. This is a neuro-developmental disorder. Negative symptoms include: flat affect, anhedonia (inability to experience pleasure), marked social aloofness/withdrawal, and the absence of florid delusions and hallucinations. Negative symptom schizophrenia tends to have an earlier and more insidious onset. As children, these people were of-ten seen as odd and aloof.

2. *Psychotic Mood Disorders*. Both mania and depression can present with poor reality testing and other psychotic symptoms.

3. *Psychosis Associated with Neurological Conditions.* Many acute metabolic and toxic states can result in a delirium. Head injury occasionally produces transient psychotic behavior and a number of degenerative diseases (e.g., Alzheimer's) can produce periods of agitated confusion. Detailed description of psychopharmacologic treatment of various neurological conditions is beyond the scope of this book. However, it is very important to distinguish such conditions from schizophrenia and mood disorders. A brief mental status exam can be helpful. It should include a test of short term memory, as well as tests for orientation and naming. Most neurologically based disorders that present with psychotic symptoms will also show gross impairment in recent/short-term memory; these abilities are relatively intact in schizophrenia. Damage to Wernicke's area (superior temporal lobe) can occasionally result in what looks like a schizophrenic reaction (language and thinking are grossly impaired). Wernicke's patients have a terrible time naming objects; people with schizophrenia and mood disorders do not. See the *Four Minute Neurological Exam* (in the MedMaster Series) for more hints on conducting a brief neurological exam. Figure 23 lists medical illnesses that may produce psychotic symptoms, and Figure 24 lists medications that may result in psychotic reactions.

NOTE: The treatment of mood disorders that present with psychotic symptoms primarily involves treating the depression (antidepressants or ECT) and adding antipsychotics to control the psychotic symptoms. Since much of this has been covered previously (Chapters 2 and 3), the focus of the following sections will be on treating schizophrenia.

Figure 23

COMMON DISEASES AND DISORDERS THAT MAY CAUSE PSYCHOSIS

- Addison's disease
- CNS infections
- CNS neoplasms
- CNS trauma
- Cushing's disease
- Delirium[1]
- Dementias[2]
- Folic acid deficiency
- Huntington's chorea

- Multiple sclerosis
- Myxedema
- Pancreatitis
- Pellagra
- Pernicious anemia
- Porphyria
- Systemic lupus erythematosis
- Temporal lobe epilepsy
- Thyrotoxicosis

---

[1]Any number of toxic/metabolic states may result in delirium

[2]Any number of dementing conditions (e.g., Alzheimer's disease) may result in psychotic symptoms.

Figure 24

COMMON DRUGS THAT MAY CAUSE PSYCHOSIS

- Sympathomimetics (e.g., cocaine and "crack," a form of almost pure cocaine, many over-the-counter cold medications)
- Antiinflamatory drugs (e.g., steroids)
- Anticholinergic drugs (e.g., antiparkinsonian drugs)
- Hallucinogenic drugs (e.g., LSD)
- L-Dopa (in schizophrenic patients)

NOTE: Older persons are often on centrally acting drugs and have less ability to tolerate their toxic effects.

Target Symptoms

It is helpful to subdivide scizophrenic symptoms into four categories: positive symptoms, disorganization symptoms, characterological traits, and negative symptoms. (See Figure 25.)

Figure 25

SCHIZOPHRENIC SYMPTOMS

POSITIVE SYMPTOMS

- Delusions and impaired thinking
- Hallucinations
- Confusion and impaired judgement
- Severe anxiety, agitation, and emotional dyscontrol

NEGATIVE SYMPTOMS

- Flat or blunted affect
- Poverty of thought (i.e., few or no thoughts and concrete thinking)
- Emptiness and anhedonia (no joy)
- Psychomotor retardation/inactivity
- Blunting of perception (e.g., insensitivity to pain)

DISORGANIZATION SYMPTOMS

- Incoherent speech
- Bizarre behavior
- Extreme confusion

CHARACTEROLOGICAL TRAITS

- Social isolation and sense of alienation
- Low self-esteem
- Social skills deficits

ANTIPSYCHOTIC MEDICATION

When Do You Prescribe Antipsychotic Medication?

Although many general practitioners treat anxiety and depressive disorders, most patients presenting with psychotic symptoms should be referred to a psychiatrist. These patients are often hard to treat. Many psychotic patients can be treated on an outpatient basis; however, hospitalization is often necessary.

Antipsychotic medications (also referred to as neuroleptics or major tranquilizers) should be started when the early signs of psychosis appear, since many times a more florid psychotic episode can be averted with appropriate early intervention.

Positive symptoms and disorganization symptoms are the primary target symptoms for treatment by antipsychotic medications. Such drugs do little to affect characterological traits or negative symptoms (with some exceptions. See page 44).

Choosing a Medication

All antipsychotic medications are equally effective in their ability to reduce positive symptoms. The choice of medication is dictated almost exclusively by the side effect profile. For a list of antipsychotic medications, see Figure 26.

Antipsychotic medications have three primary side effects which must be taken into consideration: sedation, anticholinergic (ACH), and extrapyramidal (EPS) effects.

Before choosing a medication, assess the patient's motor state. Psychotic reactions that present with marked agitation may require more sedating drugs. Use less sedating drugs for psychoses with pronounced psychomotor retardation and withdrawal. This is a general rule of thumb, but there are exceptions.

Consider anticholinergic and EPS side effects. The most common cause for relapse is poor compliance or premature discontinuation because of unpleasant side effects. The key to successful treatment rests on how well you handle side effects.

Extrapyramidal Side Effects. There are four classes of EPS:

1. *Parkinson-like Side Effects.* These include muscular rigidity, flat affect (mask-like facial expression), tremor, and bradykinesia (slowed motor responses). These symptoms need to be distinguished from the flat affect and withdrawal often seen as primary symptoms of schizophrenia. Parkinson-like side effects are often diminished by the administration of anticholinergic agents (e.g., benzotropine, trihexylphenidyl, or amantadine).

2. *Akathisia.* This is an uncontrolled sense of inner restlessness. Akathisia must be distinguished from anxiety. Often, a physician may mistake it for anxiety and increase the dose of antipsychotic, only to see a worsening of the restlessness. Akathisia can be partially alleviated by anticholinergic agents. Other

Figure 26

ANTIPSYCHOTIC MEDICATIONS

GENERIC	BRAND	DOSAGE RANGE[1]	SEDATION	EPS[2]	ACH EFFECTS[3]	EQUIVALENCE[4]
Low Potency						
chlorpromazine	Thorazine	50–1500 mg	High	+ +	+ + + +	100 mg
thioridazine	Mellaril	150–800 mg	High	+	+ + + + +	100 mg
clozapine	Clozaril	300–900 mg	High	0	+ + + + +	50 mg
mesoridazine	Serentil	50–500 mg	High	+	+ + + + +	50 mg
quetiapine	Seroquel	150–400 mg	High	+	+	50 mg
High Potency						
molindone	Moban	20–225 mg	Low	+ + +	+ + +	10 mg
perphenazine	Trilafon	8–60 mg	Mid	+ + + +	+ +	10 mg
loxapine	Loxitane	50–250 mg	Low	+ + +	+ +	10 mg
trifluoperazine	Stelazine	10–40 mg	Low	+ + + +	+ +	5 mg
fluphenazine	Prolixin[5]	3–45 mg	Low	+ + + + +	+ +	2 mg
thiothixene	Navane	10–60 mg	Low	+ + + +	+ +	5 mg
haloperidol	Haldol[5]	2–40 mg	Low	+ + + + +	+	2 mg
olanzapine	Zyprexa	5–20 mg	Mid	+	+	2 mg
pimozide	Orap	1–10 mg	Low	+ + + + +	+	2 mg
risperidone	Risperdal	4–16 mg	Low	+	+	2 mg
ziprasidone	Geodon	60–160 mg	Low	+	+ +	10 mg

[1]Usual daily oral dosage
[2]Acute: Parkinson's dystonias, akathisia. Does not reflect risk for tardive dyskinesia. All neuroleptics may cause tardive dyskinesia, except clozapine.
[3]Anticholinergic Side Effects: dry mouth, constipation, urinary retention, and blurry vision.
[4]Dose required to achieve efficacy of 100 mg chlorpromazine.
[5]Available in time-released IM format.

drugs, however, are often more successful. These include diphenhydramine, propranolol, or minor tranquilizers, such as lorazepam.

3. *Acute Dystonias.* These are muscle spasms and prolonged muscular contractions, usually of the head and neck. These can be resolved quickly with intramuscular anticholinergic agents, or treated prophylactically with oral anticholinergics.

4. *Tardive Dyskinesia (TD).* TD is generally a late onset EPS. This is a very serious and often irreversible effect of antipsychotic medication treatment. It affects about one out of 25 people treated for a period one year, and by seven

years of continuous treatment, it affects one in four (in those treated with typical antipsychotics. TD rates are lower with newer, atypical drugs). Symptoms include involuntary sucking and smacking movements of the mouth and lips, and can include chorea in the trunk and extremeties. Although various drugs have been used to reduce TD symptoms (e.g., baclofen, sodium valporate, lecithin, and benzodiazephines), there is no true cure. Treatment starts with stopping the medication. Initial worsening of the dyskinesia is expected, as the drug not only causes the syndrome but also tends to mask it. Be patient, for months if necessary, and TD will often remit. But control of severe psychosis usually outweighs the problem of TD. All patients receiving antipsychotics *must* sign an informed consent form which explains the risks of TD.

Anticholinergic Side Effects. These are the same as described in Chapter 2 on depression.

Additional Side Effects. Several potentially serious additional side affects can occur with antipsychotic medications, including agranulocytosis, impaired temperature regulations and thus increased risk of heat stroke or hypothermia, and neuroleptic malignant syndrome (a very rare syndrome that presents with fever, extrapyramidal rigidity, severe autonomic dysfunction and in some cases death. For a detailed review of this syndrome, see Pearlman, 1986). For these reasons, treatment of psychotic disorders is often more appropriately carried out by a psychiatrist.

Prescribing Treatment and What to Expect

Antipsychotic medications are generally started at low to moderate doses and titrated up until there is reduction in the more disruptive aspects of the psychotic reaction, e.g., agitation. (NOTE: Some clinicians recommend "rapid neuroleptization," i.e., very high initial doses of neuroleptics. This treatment approach is controversial and not recommended). Divided doses may be helpful initially; however, after a few days, a switch to a once-a-day bedtime dose is advisable. Dosage ranges are extremely broad and vary considerably from patient to patient. In outpatient practice, an initial starting dose might be olanzapine 2.5 mg./day or with quetiapine 100 mg./day. Inpatients are often treated at higher initial doses. See Figure 26 for dosage ranges. Antipsychotic medications must be taken each day.

Symptomatic improvement initially is seen as a decrease in arousal, emotional dyscontrol, and agitation. Poor reality testing, hallucinations, and disordered thinking may take much longer to respond. In many chronic schizophrenics, these latter symptoms may take a number of weeks to respond.

Assuming a good response, how long do you continue to treat? If the psychotic episode is a first episode, the rule of thumb is to decrease to a maintenance dose and continue to treat for one year. If the episode is a repeated episode, will probably be best to treat for two to three years before a medication-free trial is initiated. Always, owing to the risk of TD, one should treat at the lowest possible dose that provides symptomatic relief.

KEY POINTS TO COMMUNICATE TO PATIENTS

1. It is important to describe side effects to patients, especially akathisia. This side effect can be extremely unpleasant, yet often it is not spontaneously reported by patients. If it occurs and is not treated, this will greatly increase the risk of noncompliance, as well as increasing the patient's suffering. So tell patients, "You may notice an inner feeling of restlessness or nervousness. If you do, please tell me. Do not just discontinue the medication. Most side effects can be treated."

2. Schizophrenia is a relapsing disorder and it is extremely important to keep taking medication even if things seem fine. Premature discontinuation is the primary cause of relapse.

3. The total length of treatment is likely to be at least one year and often longer for more chronic schizophrenia.

4. Antipsychotic medications are not addictive.

5. You should avoid prolonged exposure to high temperatures and sunlight (some antipsychotics have photosensitivity as a side effect).

6. Avoid amphetamines, cocaine, and L-Dopa because these drugs almost always exacerbate psychoses.

7. You and your relatives need to know about the risk of TD (and sign appropriate consent forms.)

Treatment-Resistant Schizophrenic Disorders

There are three main reasons why schizophrenic patients may not respond to antipsychotic medication:

1. *Poor compliance.* Often this is due to the unpleasant side effects. Many times patient education and proper medical management of side effects resolve the problem. Sometimes, patients simply forget to take their medication. In such cases, treatment with time-released intramuscular forms of antipsychotics can be helpful. Additionally, involving the family in treatment can significantly enhance compliance.

Figure 27

DECISION TREE FOR DIAGNOSIS AND TREATMENT
OF PSYCHOSIS

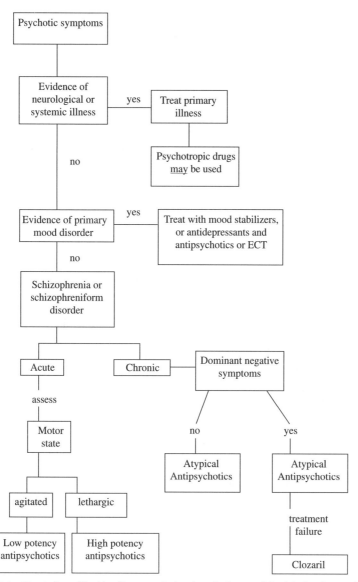

Note: Due to favorable side effects, atypical antipsychotics are advised (unless long-acting
IM antipsychotics are warranted).

43

2. *Inadequate doses.* Blood levels can be monitored and doses increased as indicated.

3. Negative symptom schizophrenics may have a different underlying pathophysiology and often do not respond well to traditional antipsychotics. These patients are hard to treat.

Several, newer antipsychotic medications have shown promise in treating the negative (as well as positive) symptoms of schizophrenia. The first is clozapine (brand name Clozaril). Clozapine became available in the United States in 1990. This medication is considered to be an atypical antipsychotic agent; its pharmacologic profile is different than other existing antipsychotics. The first important feature is that initial trials show it to be effective in treating many schizophrenic patients who have failed to respond to standard antipsychotic drugs. This includes a number of patients that presented with negative symptoms (as well as other treatment-resistant schizophrenics). The second important and unique feature is the virtual lack of acute extrapyramidal symptoms and few reported cases of tardive dyskinesia. This medication does have two significant potential side effects: (1) The incidence of clozapine-induced agranulocytosis (a potentially fatal blood dyscrasia) is between 1 and 2%, as compared to the incidence seen in other antipsychotics (about 0.1%). This problem, however, is proving to be avoidable through a mandatory hematological monitoring program (weekly medication dispensing occurs only if the patient's white blood cell count is normal). Since implementing this program, there have been no fatalities in the 15 cases of clozapine-related agranulocytosis reported in the United States. If there is a low WBC count, medication is immediately discontinued and, to date, all such cases have been reversible. (2) A second troublesome side effect is a fairly high incidence of seizures (about 1–2% at low doses and 5% at higher doses). Despite these problematic features, clozapine appears to represent an important breakthrough in the management of otherwise treatment-resistant schizophrenic disorders.

The newest additions to the "atypical" list are risperidone, olanzapine, quetiapine, and ziprasidone, providing additional options for treating both positive and negative psychotic symptoms with a much more benign side effect profile when compared to standard antipsychotics. These medications do not have the high incidence of agranulocytosis seen with clozapine.

Common Treatment Errors to Avoid

- Akathisia (extreme inner sense of restlessness) is a very common side effect that is quite uncomfortable and a primary cause for patient-initiated discontinuation. Remarkably, many schizophrenic patients will not spontaneously complain of this side effect, but simply discontinue. It is therefore important to inquire specifically about the presence of akathisia during follow-up visits
- Be especially watchful for early signs of tardive dyskinesia. Early signs can be elicited by having the patient lay his/her arms on lap while seated,

extending the fingers in a relaxed, downward position over the knees. Note: for the presence of spontaneous, purposeless, jerking movements of the fingers

- Antipsychotics often produce significant emotional blunting and apathy or Parkinsonian symptoms which may be mis-identified as negative symptoms (in such cases, raising the dose will likely exacerbate the side effects)

Books to Recommend to Patients and Their Families

Torrey, E.F. (2001). *Surviving Schizophrenia: A Family Manual*, Harper and Row Publishers.

Mueser, K. and Gingerich, S. (1994). *Coping with Schizophrenia: A Guide for Families*, New Harbinger, Oakland.

Chapter 6   Miscellaneous Disorders

In this chapter we would like to briefly discuss six additional disorders for which psychotropic medications can be useful.

OBSESSIVE-COMPULSIVE DISORDER

Major Clinical Features

The major features of this disorder are recurring obsessions (persistent, intrusive, troublesome thoughts or impulses that are recognized by the patient as senseless) and/or compulsions (repetitive behaviors or rituals enacted in response to an obsession, e.g., repeatedly checking to see if doors are locked, compulsive hand washing, or counting). In order to meet the criteria for obsessive compulsive disorder, the obsessions and/or compulsions must create significant distress or be time consuming enough to interfere with normal routines.

Medication Treatment

Treatments of choice include the use of serotinergic antidepressants (see below) often in combination with behavior therapy. Without behavior therapy, relapse is likely with discontinuation. Thus, chronic medication treatment is generally necessary.

Figure 28

NAME				
Generic	Brand	Dose Range	Sedation	ACH Effects
clomipramine	Anafranil	150–300 mg	Hi	Hi
fluoxetine	Prozac[1]	20–80 mg	Low	None
sertraline	Zoloft[1]	50–200 mg	Low	None
paroxetine	Paxil[1]	20–50 mg	Low	Low
fluvoxamine	Luvox	50–300 mg	Low	Low
citalopram	Celexa	10–60 mg	Low	None
escitalopram	Lexapro	5–20 mg	Low	None

[1]often higher doses are required to control obsessive-compulsive symptoms than the doses generally used to treat depression.

BORDERLINE PERSONALITY DISORDER

Major Clinical Features

Borderline personality disorders constitute a very heterogeneous group of individuals that suffer from long-term emotional instability. As a group they are characterized by the following features: a pattern of chaotic, unstable relationships, significant emotional lability, impulsiveness (e.g., self-mutilation, suicide attempts, substance abuse, very poor frustration tolerance, sexual promiscuity), anger control problems (e.g. pronounced irritability, temper tantrums, etc.), a tendency to develop significant bouts of anxiety and depression, and chronic feelings of emptiness. Some borderline patients can develop transient psychotic symptoms (that usually remit within hours to days). These patients are prone to any number of major psychiatric syndromes in addition to what is a very stable, chronic pattern of maladaptive functioning in life.

Medication Treatment

Although there is increasing data to suggest an underlying biologic cause in many of these patients, it is generally felt that the basic disorder is an outgrowth of significant early, maladaptive psychological development (e.g. severe child neglect). Psychotropic medications in no way treat the basic personality disorder, however, medications can be used to treat particular target symptoms.

Not all borderline patients are alike, and for treatment purposes, the following subgroups can be delineated to provide guidelines for choosing medications. The subgroups are defined by the presence of a dominant symptom picture. Note: investigators to date have found that minor tranquilizers generally are not indicated in the treatment of borderline personality disorder. These patients often experience an increased degree of emotional dyscontrol/disinhibition with minor tranquilizers, and are at high risk for abusing such drugs.

Figure 29

SUB-GROUPS	DRUGS OF CHOICE
1. Impulsivity/Anger Control Problems	Serotonergic antidepressants, e.g. fluoxetine, sertraline
2. Schizotypal (peculiar thinking, transient psychosis)	Low doses of antipsychotic medications e.g. 2.5 mg olanzapine, 1 mg. risperidone
3. Extreme sensitivity to rejection/ being alone	Serotonergic antidepressants
4. Emotional instability	Lithium, divalproex, atypical antipsychotics

ATTENTION DEFICIT DISORDER[1]

Attention deficit disorder (ADD)[2] affects between 3–5% of children. It is now widely held that this disorder is largely due to a neurochemical disturbance (likely involving dysregulation of dopamine and/or norepinephrine in the frontal cortex).

Recent longitudinal/follow-up studies indicate that as many as 70% of ADD children continue to exhibit symptoms well into adolescence and adult life, thus suggesting that potentially 2–3% of the adult population experience ADD symptoms. The major symptoms of ADD are outlined in Figure 30.

Figure 30

SYMPTOMS OF ADD

■ Impulsivity, e.g. acting before thinking, quick responses, poor judgement

■ Difficulties in feeling motivated

■ Impaired abilities for attention and concentration; distractibility

■ Difficulties organizing tasks and activities

■ Restlessness and "hyperactivity"

■ Impaired emotional controls

■ Associated features:

　　Learning disabilities

　　Low self-esteem

With age and maturation 30% of ADD kids "grow out of it" and exhibit no ongoing symptoms. The remaining 70% tend to see a gradual reduction in restlessness and "hyperactivity" although other core ADD symptoms remain.

ADD kids and teenagers often encounter considerable social/peer rejection and academic failure. Self-esteem problems and frank clinical depression are not uncommon. Rates of substance abuse in *un*treated ADD adolescents are high (probably best seen as an attempt to medicate-away feelings of sadness and inadequacy).

The discussion of pharmacologic treatment of ADD with children and young teens is beyond the scope of this book (the reader is referred to an excellent text by Kutcher, 2002). Older adolescent and adult ADD clients can be very successfully treated with psychotropic medications (success rates approaching 90%).

The mainstay of pharmacologic treatment of ADD is the use of stimulants (See Figure 31). Please note that the three fast-acting stimulants listed (methylphenidate, amphetamine, and dextroamphetamine) can become drugs of abuse in those predisposed to chemical dependency. Thus caution should be exercised in treating patients with a substance abuse history. (Note: studies of ADD children, adolescents and adults *without* a personal or family history of substance abuse, show no

---

[1]Adapted from Preston, Lucas and O'Neal, 1995.

[2]Also referred to as Attention Deficit/Hyperactivity Disorder (ADHD).

Figure 31

MEDICATIONS USED TO TREAT ADD

GENERIC	BRAND	DAILY DOSES
Stimulants		
methylphenidate	Ritalin	5–50 mg.
methylphenidate	Concerta	18–36 mg.
methylphenidate	Metadate	10–40 mg.
dextroamphetamine	Dexedrine	5–40 mg.
pemoline	Cylert	37.5–112.5 mg.
d- and l-amphetamine	Adderall	5–40 mg.
Antidepressants		
imipramine	Tofranil	75–300 mg.
buproprion, SR	Wellbutrin, SR	150–300 mg.

tendency to abuse these stimulant drugs.) And the abuse potential does not occur with pemoline or the antidepressants listed in Figure 31.

Because ADD (in adults) is almost always a life-long condition, prolonged medication treatment is the rule rather than the exception.

AGGRESSION

Major Clinical Features

Marked aggression (including irritability, hostility, violence), whether chronic or episodic, is seen in a number of psychiatric and neurologic disorders, including those listed in Figure 32.

Figure 32

PSYCHIATRIC DISORDERS PRESENTING WITH SYMPTOMS OF AGGRESSION

- A.D.D./ADHD
- Anti-Social Personality Disorder
- Borderline Personality Disorder
- Conduct Disorder
- Delirium
- Dementias
- Depression
- Explosive Disorder
- Iatrogenic, e.g. steroid use
- Mania
- Mental Retardation
- Paranoid Disorder
- Post-concussion syndrome
- Schizophrenia
- Substance use disorders
- Temporal lobe epilepsy

In most cases, the preferred strategy is to treat the primary disorder (e.g. antipsychotics with schizophrenics). Beyond this, certain medication treatment options exist (See Figure 33). However, it is important to note that no single treatment for aggressive behavior has been devised that has a high rate of success. The clinician must consider side effects of all potential agents and then proceed with a systematic trial of available medications until one proves to be helpful. Regretfully, severe aggression continues to be a target symptom that is very difficult to treat.

Figure 33

MEDICATION OPTIONS IN THE TREATMENT OF AGGRESSION

- Anticonvulsants (e.g. divalproex)
- Antipsychotics
- Beta blockers (e.g. propranolol)
- Buspirone
- Clonidine
- Lithium
- SSRIs

EATING DISORDERS

Eating disorders are generally categorized as follows: bulimia (periodic binge eating following by purging) and anorexia nervosa (intense fear of becoming fat and a refusal to maintain healthy, age-appropriate body weight).

Unfortunately, anorexia nervosa, which can often be a life-threatening illness, has a poor response rate to a host of standard psychotopic medications. It has been treated experimentally with the opiate antagonist, naltrexone. Because it is potentially a very severe disorder, a referral to a psychiatrist or a specialized eating disorders program is almost always warranted.

Bulimia, however, often is responsive to treatment with antidepressants (even in the absence of depressive symptoms). The clinician should treat bulimia much in the same way as he/she treats depression (i.e., with regard to dosing, length of treatment, etc.). All antidepressants lower seizure threshold and this can be especially problematic in this metabolically unstable group. Thus caution is warranted (especially if treating with maprotiline or immediate release bupropion).

POST-TRAUMATIC STRESS DISORDER

Post-traumatic stress disorder (P.T.S.D.) may be seen in the aftermath of recently occurring severe stressful events or can present in a chronic form which continues for many years after traumatic experiences (the latter is often seen in individuals who experienced very severe abuse as children). The symptoms of P.T.S.D. vary, and can include the following: generalized anxiety, panic attacks, depression, transient psychotic symptoms, intrusive symptoms (intense unwanted memories, flashbacks or nightmares) and states of emotional numbness.

The treatment of choice for P.T.S.D. is psychotherapy. Psychotropic medication treatment may be helpful in reducing certain target symptoms (treatments for panic and depressive symptoms follow general guidelines for these conditions). Additionally, three symptoms of P.T.S.D. warrant specific comments.

Transient psychotic symptoms often respond to a *short course* of antipsychotic agents. Often, the doses required are somewhat lower than that generally required to treat schizophrenia. Intrusive symptoms have been treated with a host of psychiatric medications. To date, the best outcomes are achieved with SSRI antidepressants. It should be noted that often high doses may be required (e.g. 60–80 mg fluoxetine or 200 mg. sertraline). Although no specific medication targets emotional numbing, often once intrusive symptoms are diminished, there is a corresponding decrease in the frequency and intensity of numbness (and related symptoms such as dissociation, depersonalization and derealization).

Books to Recommend to Patients and Their Families

Obsessive-Compulsive
Rapoport, J. L. (1989). *The Boy Who Couldn't Stop Washing,* Signet: New York.

Steketee, G. and White, K. (1990). *When Once is Not Enough: Help for Obsessive-Compulsives.* New Harbinger, Oakland, CA.

ADD
Barkley, R. and Murphy, K. (1998). *Attention Deficit Hyperactivity Disorder,* Guilford Press, New York.

Borderline Personality Disorder
Kreisman, J. and Krauss, H. (1988). *I Hate You—Don't Leave Me: Understanding Borderline Personality Disorder,* Price Stern: New York.

Mason, P. and Kreger, R. (1998). *Stop Walking On Eggshells,* New Harbinger, Oakland, CA.

Aggression
Potter-Efron, R. (1989). *Angry All the Time,* New Harbinger, Oakland, CA.

Eating Disorders
Sandbek, T. (1993). *The Deadly Diet: Recovering from Anorexia and Bulimia* (Second Edition), New Harbinger, Oakland, CA.

Post-traumatic Stress Disorder
Matsakis, A. (1992). *I Can't Get Over It: A Handbook for Trauma Survivors,* New Harbinger, Oakland, CA.

Greist, J.H. et al. (2000). *Post-Traumatic Stress Disorder: A Guide,* Madison Institute of Medicine, Madison, Wisconsin.

A General Reference for Clients to Help Them Understand the Process of Psychotherapy and the Role of Medications

Preston, J., Varzos, N., and Liebert, D. (2000). *Make Every Session Count,* New Harbinger, Oakland, CA.

Chapter 7   Non-Response and "Breakthrough Symptoms" Algorithms

When the diagnosis is made and treatment initiated, if there is a failure to respond to treatment then the following algorithm can provide a strategy for re-evaluation:

NON-RESPONSE CHECKLIST

1. Re-evaluate the initial diagnosis

2. Rule out co-existing medical illness

3. Rule out substance abuse (which often interferes with the metabolism of psychotropic medications and/or exacerbates psychiatric symptoms)

4. Rule out medication induced psychiatric symptoms (e.g. antihypertensives causing depression)

5. Has there been an adequate trial? This always assumes:

    a. Adequate dose (may necessitate monitoring blood levels)

    b. Adequate duration of time (remember, most psychotropics require several weeks of treatment before the onset of symptom reduction)

    c. Compliance (notoriously poor among psychiatric patients). Monitor side effects.

6. Rule out drug-drug interactions that may affect pharmacokinetics

7. Psychological and psychosocial issues are not being adequately addressed (refer for psychotherapy)

8. The patient may be on the wrong class of medications and/or require augmentation.

Not infrequently a patient has a positive initial response to treatment and later experiences a return of symptoms. In such instances the clinician can assess the following:

UNEXPLAINED RELAPSE CHECKLIST

1. Recent onset or increase in substance use/abuse

2. Sleep disturbance has become more pronounced due to increased stress, physical pain, and/or substance use (e.g. caffeine). Sleep deprivation *always* increases psychiatric symptoms.

3. Failure to comply with medication treatment

4. Significant increases in psychosocial stressors

5. Changes in underlying metabolic factors and/or neurobiologic changes (e.g. impaired hepatic or renal functioning, recent head injury, menopause)

6. Tolerance for the psychotropic medication may have developed (although this is rare).

7. Rule out an underlying medical disorder.

Chapter 8   Case Examples

In this chapter we will present a number of case examples which illustrate commonly encountered clinical issues and problems (with suggested solutions and strategies). Although general principles are helpful in initiating treatment, in a real sense each case is unique and somewhat of an experiment. Accurate diagnostic assessment and a review of the patient's personal and health status (e.g., age, medical problems, prescription drugs being taken, etc.) will certainly help determine initial psychotropic medication choices. However, beyond this starting point, the clinician must track patient response closely to monitor for compliance, side effect problems and eventual symptomatic improvement.

In managed care, HMO, and family practice settings, compliance problems abound. This is due to five common factors: a) inadequate patient education regarding the medication, b) the emergence of side effects and c) the frequent problems of demoralization and feelings of hopelessness (i.e., many psychiatric patients come to the clinician in a state of despair and pessimism. When psychiatric medications do not rapidly provide symptom improvement or unpleasant side effects occur, many patients abruptly stop taking medications or drop out of treatment), d) inadequate follow-up, and e) general aversion to/fear of taking medications, especially psychiatric medications, for a variety of psychosocially and philosophically based reasons, which the patient often will not share spontaneously. Frequently such patients deteriorate and re-emerge later either in a more severe psychological state, or are seen and treated for a host of stress-related somatic symptoms.

It is our opinion that more time spent initially in diagnosis and treatment followup can contribute significantly to successful treatment outcomes. Hopefully this chapter will highlight common treatment complications and suggested action strategies.

In the treatment of anxiety and depressive disorders, the "rule of threes" seems to apply. About one-third of patients are fairly uncomplicated and can be treated successfully with psychotropic medications, brief supportive counseling and the support offered by social networks (family, friends, churches, support groups). A second third of patients are more challenging. These people experience medication-related problems (e.g., side effect problems, inadequate response to standard regimens or failure to respond to first-line medications) and/or are in need of more intensive psychotherapy where treatment by a professional therapist is indicated. Yet despite these added challenges, this group can generally be managed quite successfully.*

---

*Note: In the United States, family practice and other non-psychiatric physicians treat the majority of people seeking help for depressive and anxiety disorders, writing 69% of all prescription for antidepressants and 90% of all prescriptions for antianxiety medications.

The remaining third are significantly more difficult to treat and most often must have medications managed by a psychiatrist as well as being involved in psychotherapy.

The treatment of bipolar and psychotic disorders is considerably more difficult owing to three factors: a) these severe mental illnesses often require inpatient treatment, b) the medications used can have more problematic and serious side effects (often requiring more monitoring of the patient's medical status) and c) the medication regimen often is more complicated. For these reasons, although some relatively uncomplicated and treatment-responsive bipolar and psychotic patients can be and are treated in primary care settings, a referral to a psychiatrist is usually necessary.

CASE A: A Case of Major Depression

Background and Presenting Problems: Mr. E. is a 62 year old retired draftsman. He has suffered for 20+ years from rather severe arthritis. He takes over-the-counter pain medication and currently is on no prescribed medication. Beyond the arthritis, Mr. E. is in good health. Characterologically, he can be seen as a rigid, obsessional man who has had few close friends aside from business colleagues and his wife of 35 years. He is a stamp collector and since his retirement two years ago he has become progressively isolated and withdrawn.

Mr. E. comes to you complaining of problems with his "nerves" and insomnia. His grooming is adequate, but he appears to be quite fatigued. He reports that problems have developed over the past three months ever since his wife confessed to having a "one night fling" with an old boyfriend while she was visiting relatives out of town. She promises that the affair is not on-going, but he worries almost constantly about her "leaving me" and harbors significant anger towards her.

Mr. E's symptoms include: irritability, an almost total loss of the capacity for experiencing pleasure, fatigue, an inner sense of restlessness, a 15 pound weight loss over the past three months, suicidal ideas, loss of libido and a sleep disturbance (restless sleep almost every night and early-morning awakening 5 nights out of 7 during the past six weeks).

Diagnosis Issues: The initial impressions are that Mr. E. has a major depression. (Because of no previous episodes of depression or mania, it is considered to be a single-episode, unipolar depression.) Although clearly this depression is "reactive" (i.e., in response to a significant psychosocial stressor), the symptom picture reveals the presence of physiological symptoms (see pg. 5) which suggest a neurochemical dysregulation and indicate that he is a candidate for antidepressants.

Initial Medication Treatment Issues and Decisions: Although Mr. E. reports an inner sense of restlessness, he is quite fatigued and his overall motor state is retarded. Thus it makes sense to choose a more stimulating antidepressant. You choose fluoxetine. Mr. E. is prescribed a 10 mg. q.d. dose, is given proper patient education underscoring two points: a) the medication will take 2–4 weeks to yield symptomatic improvement and he needs to be patient and take the medicine as prescribed, and b) be sure to call if he notices any significant side effects. (He is told the most common side effects which may occur with this medication.) After one week you increase the dose to 20 mg. q.d. Two days later, Mr. E. calls to say that he is feeling "jittery." You instruct him to reduce the dose to 10 mg. q.d. for a week. You ask him to touch base with you by phone in the next day or so. Upon follow-up, the jitteriness has disappeared and he reports no other side effects. After a week on 10 mg. q.d., he is instructed again to increase to 20 mg. q.d.; he does so this time without noticeable side effects.

Points to Underscore:

- Minor side effect problems are common with all antidepressants, and most can be managed by dosage adjustment. As patients tolerate lower doses, the doctor can then gradually titrate the dose up into the therapeutic range.
- Patient education and close doctor-patient communication are the keys to initiating treatment dealing with early emergent problems.

Course of Treatment: Let's consider three possible outcomes.

Scenario One: By day 18 of treatment, now on 20 mg. q.d. for nine days, Mr. E. *begins* to report less daytime fatigue, somewhat better sleep and reduced irritability. He continues on the same dose, and by day 40 almost all major depressive symptoms have resolved. He still has on-going issues with his wife (for which they are in couples counseling with their minister), but core depressive symptoms are resolved. You instruct Mr. E. to continue on the antidepressant at the same dose for an additional six months before discontinuing (a highly recommended strategy to reduce the likelihood of acute relapse). The medication is discontinued six months later and he remains asymptomatic.

Scenario Two: By day 30 Mr. E. reports only a slight improvement in his sleep, but otherwise remains quite depressed. At this point it is very important to ask or review a number of key questions:

- Is he taking the medication as prescribed?
- Is he abusing alcohol or illicit drugs? (Concurrent and often unreported alcohol abuse is a *very common* reason for inadequate response to antidepressants.)
- Have psychosocial stressors increased?
- Although he reported that, aside from arthritis, his general health status was good, could there be an undiagnosed medical condition contributing to his depressive symptoms (e.g., hypothyroidism)? An old saying is "Dogs can have fleas *and* ticks"; always consider the possibility of symptoms related to life stressors *and* coexisting medical conditions.

If all questions have been addressed and none of these factors appear to be contributing to his lack of response, the next step will be to increase the medication dose (if and only if Mr. E. tolerates side effects).

In this scenario we will assume that he does tolerate an increase to 40 mg. q.d. of fluoxetine. After seven days on the new dose, he begins to respond positively.

Within a few weeks, all depressive symptoms resolve. He is then maintained on the *same* 40 mg. q.d. dose for six months before discontinuation.

Scenario Three: As above, after an increase to 40 mg. q.d., Mr. E. fails to show clinical improvement. He is maintained on the dose for two weeks. You decide to increase again to 60 mg., but after two weeks there is still little improvement. At this point there are two options: a) augment or b) switch to a different class of medication.

Scenario Three - A: You decide to add lithium 300 mg. b.i.d to the fluoxetine and within two weeks, Mr. E. begins to show the first signs of symptomatic improvement.

Scenario Three - B: Mr. E. either cannot tolerate lithium or fails the augmentation trial. You decide to switch to another class of antidepressant. Thus you decide to switch to bupropion, SR. (Since fluoxetine is a serotonergic drug, the most reasonable choice for second-line treatment is an antidepressant that affects norepinephrine.) You allow for a one week no-drug wash out and then start bupropion, SR, beginning with a low dose, 100 mg. q.d.

In order to avoid or minimize initial side effect problems, it is advisable to start with low doses, gradually titrating up every 4 days, as tolerated by the patient.

The dose of bupropion, SR is gradually increased during the first week until it reaches the therapeutic range (i.e., 150 mg) (Note: since Mr. E. is 62 years old, general metabolic activity, as with most older people, is slowed in the liver, and thus may benefit from lower doses, e.g., 100 mg. q.d. However, almost without exception, younger and middle-aged adults require doses within the therapeutic range (see figure 5). As doses are increased, the clinician always monitors two variables: signs of clinical improvement and side effects. In the scenario, Mr. E. was able to reach a dose of 150 mg. of bupropion, SR by day 7, tolerating the medication well. By day 14 he began to respond.

Had he failed the 150 mg. trial, several options still exist:

- Progressively increase the dose of bupropion, SR up to a maximum of 300 mg. q.d. (if necessary and if tolerated).
- Take a bupropion, SR blood level to assure that it is within the therapeutic range.
- Augment with lithium.
- Switch classes of medications to either an MAO inhibitor (after an appropriate 2 week wash out of bupropion) or the antidepressant, venlafaxine.
- Electroconvulsive therapy is a final option if all other treatments fail and/or if his condition deteriorates and suicidal impulses intensify.

Throughout treatment the clinician should continue to monitor for the presence of alcohol use/abuse, medical problems, and the use of other prescription drugs. And it is *always* important to consider psychotherapy as an important aspect of treatment, especially in cases such as that of Mr. E., where psychosocial and interpersonal issues play such an important role in the genesis of his depression.

CASE B: A Case of Bipolar Illness

Mr. M. is a 22 year-old college student brought to you by his parents after a two-week history of marked change in his usual behavior. At first, he began staying up later and getting up earlier. Although his parents assumed he was studying for his impending final examinations, they were puzzled by his high energy and enthusiasm in the morning since he was usually a slow starter, especially if he did not get a good night's sleep. Concern began when they discovered that he was not, in fact, studying at all, but was working on a new computer program that would make him a millionaire. He was vague on details and brushed aside objections that he had little knowledge of computer equipment and became irritable and demanding when they questioned the wisdom and reality of this behavior. He had always been a reasonable and somewhat conservative individual. In addition, he seemed to talk incessantly and without any interest in input from others, although attempted input by others would often send him off on a tangential line of discourse. Concern turned to alarm, anger and embarrassment when he made inappropriate sexual comments to one of his mother's friends who had come to visit. The patient came for a consultation only with the firm insistence of his parents, and only to make them happy since he felt nothing was wrong with his behavior.

A history confirms the patient's prior apparent excellent adjustment without psychiatric consultation and a negative recent physical exam and full chemistry screen prior to his tryout for a baseball team.

The patient denies drug use, and his parents had found no evidence of drug use. A urine screen for drugs of abuse is obtained and confirms no drugs.

An uncle had had several episodes of erratic and irresponsible behavior, leading to financial problems and divorce, but he was the black sheep of the family and was a heavy abuser of alcohol, which the family had blamed for his misfortunes.

At this point the family practitioner should remind himself or herself of the following points:

- The diagnosis of manic or hypomanic states is relatively easy as it is dramatic and unlikely to be confused with other conditions *provided* drug abuse is ruled out, especially stimulants.
- Bipolar disorder is often complicated in its long term course by associated difficulties, especially of a psychosocial nature, and drug regimens for certain variant forms of the illness. It is, therefore, usually best left to the care of a psychiatrist. This is especially true if the illness has been present for some time, is rapidly cycling, or if the patient is on other medications.
- The difficulty in treating manic or hypomanic states at the outset is usually in enlisting cooperation and compliance with treatment. A good rapport or relationship with the patient is critical; working with and through the family is often critical as well.
- Do not be misled by the ability of patients to hold it together for a doctor's visit. Those patients who are clearly manic and who exhibit the classic signs on mental status exams should be referred immediately to a psychiatrist,

except for those rare patients with insight and who present themselves for treatment (and these usually have a history of prior episodes).

• Lithium carbonate is the drug of choice. Failure of the patient to respond to lithium should trigger a referral to, or consultation with, a psychiatrist.

In this case, you are fortunate in that the patient has seen you in the past for physical exams and minor medical problems, and you have had good rapport. With professional concern and authoritative directness, but without condescension, you tell the patient that while he may not agree, it is your medical opinion that he has a medical condition that is well known and produces the kind of symptoms he has been having. You may want to review the reported behavior and your own observations if they have included hypomanic or manic behavior. Do not do this in an exhortatory way but in an analytical manner which arrives at your recommendation for treatment. You then educate the patient about the major side effects of lithium and get an informed consent. If the patient attempts to minimize or escape by declaring "he'll think about it," recognize with him that you cannot make him take the medication, of course, but that you really think it is important for him to take the lithium and proffer the prescription.

Assuming compliance, you begin lithium 300 mgs. b.i.d., with meals and measure the serum lithium level in two days on a stat basis. If the lithium level is below 1.0 meq/L increase to 300 mg. t.i.d., and again measure the serum lithium level in two days. At each visit inquire about side effects and reassure him, if they are in a tolerable range, that they are not dangerous and will lessen in the near future. The maintenance goal is 1.0 meq/L but side effects may necessitate a compromise. Levels below 0.5 meq/L are generally considered subtherapeutic. Continue to raise the dose by 300 mg. q.d., and measure the lithium level every two days until it is 1.0 meq/L. If the patient fails to respond within two weeks, consult a psychiatrist.

If the patient responds beautifully, he should remain on maintenance therapy indefinitely. A patient will rarely comply with this but monthly checks over the next several months encourage the patient to share with you his feelings about having a chronic mental disorder and the need to have chronic treatment; answer those questions which you can. As long as the patient remains in treatment, he will need periodic blood tests for lithium, TSH (lithium occasionally produces hypothyroidism, a serious problem when untreated but easily treated) and creatinine (lithium is excreted by the kidney and decreased renal clearance could lead to lithium toxicity). This should be done usually about every three months. In general, proceed as in case C.

CASE C: Another Case of Bipolar Disorder

A 45 year-old married housewife with a history of three episodes of mania and two mild depressions during her twenties presents with a request to continue her lithium and to get "blood checks." She has been quite stable on lithium since beginning treatment around the age of 28, experiencing only two mild elated periods. She is in good health except for diabetes mellitus, controlled with diet alone. The patient has been quite compliant with treatment and states that her husband is fully informed of her condition and is able to identify her mood swings, often before she does. A review of her prior medical records indicates the presence of clear criteria for bipolar disorder including one brief hospitalization for the second episode of elation during which she was engaged in some sexually promiscuous behavior which was embarrassing and quite out of character. Her depressions were significant but not associated with suicidal behavior. She had been responsive to lithium but stopped it after leaving the hospital. She quickly responded to lithium again on the third episode of elation, obviating the need for hospitalization. The records also revealed that a lithium level of 0.8meq/L controlled her symptoms adequately, but that higher levels produced some shakiness in her hands, which she found annoying. She was quite satisfied with her care, but had recently moved to the area because of her husband's transfer secondary to a promotion. The only psychiatrist in the area was not taking new patients.

Increasingly, the family practitioner will be sought out for medication maintenance by already diagnosed and regulated patients who have moved, changed insurance coverage, or whose psychiatrist has retired or moved. Once again, the history should be reviewed and only those cases which are uncomplicated (see above points to keep in mind) should be accepted.

The follow-up interval is arbitrary, but every three months is adequate in uncomplicated situations. An elevated TSH should be treated by thyroid replacement. An elevation in lithium or creatinine levels should trigger an evaluation of kidney function. Symptoms of lithium toxicity should be reviewed with the patient and her husband, with instructions to report in if these toxic symptoms are noted at any time. These brief routine visits not only establish the rapport so vital to treatment of episodes, but they also allow the practitioner to establish a baseline mental status to compare with changes produced by a mood shift. Blood for lab studies is best drawn in the morning before eating (fluids are permitted, but milk or cream should be avoided) and before the morning lithium dose. Finally, any increase in frequency of episodes, even mild ones, should trigger psychiatric consultation.

CASE D: A Case of Acute Situational Anxiety

Background and Presenting Problems: Mrs. M. is a 47 year-old bank executive. She is married and has three teenage children. Her history is one of reasonably good adjustment and no episodes of prior psychiatric symptoms. Two weeks ago her husband was diagnosed with malignant melanoma. He is undergoing treatment and the prognosis is fairly positive. However, since the diagnosis Mrs. M. has experienced a considerable amount of anxiety and worry. She can hardly put her husband's illness out of her mind, and throughout the day she ruminates.

Her ability to concentrate at work has become noticeably impaired. She has frequent waves of nervousness in which she trembles and experiences a mild degree of shortness of breath and tachycardia. She also reports difficulties falling asleep (requires 1½–2 hours to go to sleep, although when asleep she is able to sleep through the night). She is in good health and currently is taking no prescription medications.

Diagnostic Issues: Given this presentation several important questions come to mind:

- Is there any evidence that she is clinically depressed? Many patients that initially appear to have anxiety symptoms are, in fact, depressed. This differential diagnosis is important. So you question her about important symptoms such as: self-esteem, anhedonia, decreased libido, fatigue, early morning awakening, etc.
- Is she using/abusing drugs (being especially concerned with determining the amount of caffeine use)?
- Are there any undiagnosed medical problems (remember, fleas *and* ticks) e.g., hyperthyroidism?

She is sad, especially when imagining that her husband could die. However, she does not exhibit severe or entrenched symptoms of major depression. She is not abusing drugs and, in fact, is in good health. You diagnosis is an adjustment disorder with anxiety symptoms (i.e., stress-related anxiety).

Initial Medication Treatment Issues and Decisions: Brief counseling or psychotherapy is the treatment of choice for this type of disorder. Medications can also be a helpful adjunct. You tell Mrs. M. that her symptoms are understandable given her life circumstances, but you also acknowledge that the impaired concentration at work and her insomnia certainly are problematic, and *short term* medication treatment may be helpful. One very important question must be addressed prior to initiating treatment: Is there any personal or family history of alcoholism or drug abuse? If so, she should be considered *at risk* for misuse or abuse of benzodiazepines. Assuming she denies any reported history of substance abuse, she is prescribed one of the following: a) a low dose benzodiazepine for occasional daytime use (e.g., lorazepam 0.5 mg. b.i.d, prn), if the target symptoms are daytime anxiety and impaired concentration or, b) a low to moderate dose of a hypnotic (e.g., temazepam, 15 mg. q.h.s., prn) if you choose to treat the insomnia.

Mrs. M. is told that this medication is for short-term use only (probably 1–4 weeks). Should her stressors and symptoms continue beyond this point, it will probably be necessary for her to be in counseling and to be reevaluated. If she is using these medications appropriately and circumstances warrant it, continued treatment beyond 4 weeks may be indicated and helpful. You are especially alert to monitor two issues as treatment progresses:

- Many patients may not fully benefit from very low doses of benzodiazepines, and a dosage increase may be appropriate. However, overuse of medications or ongoing requests/demands for higher doses, should alert the clinician to the possibility of benzodiazepine abuse.

- Should Mrs. M. require daily use of a benzodiazepine for more than 3 or 4 weeks, the clinician must consider that dependence can develop. Tolerance generally does not develop for the antianxiety effects of benzodiazepines; however, habituation that can occur neurophysiologically and can (and often does) result in withdrawal symptoms if the medication is abruptly discontinued. Thus, when you determine that it is time to discontinue, this should be done gradually. A wise approach is to take at least one month to progressively wean Mrs. M. from her antianxiety medication (if she has been on it for more than one month).

Once again, especially in cases of reactive distress, keep in mind that counseling or psychotherapy are very important, in addition to psychotropic medications, patient education, and general reassurance.

CASE E: A Case of Panic Disorder

Background and Presenting Problems: Ms. B. is a 32 year-old, single vocational counselor. Although she has not had a history of major psychiatric symptoms, she did have several bouts of "nervousness," each time in response to significant life transitions. The first of these was in high school when her family moved to a new state. It was a difficult adjustment for her. She missed her old friends a lot, and for 2–3 months felt extremely anxious. She was often afraid to leave the house, although she did manage to go to school despite her distress. She also felt afraid when her parents left her at home alone for an evening. After several months, her anxiety subsided. The second episode was when she went to college. She attended a school some 200 miles away from her home town. She again felt very anxious, developed some type of undiagnosable stomach pain, and eventually dropped out. Ms. B. moved home and enrolled in a local community college, and her anxiety subsided.

After graduation from college, she secured a job with a company in her home town and has maintained fairly close contact with her parents over the years.

Six weeks ago her father suffered a heart attack. He was in critical condition for two days, but progressively recovered and currently is doing well. However, the day after his heart attack Ms. B. experienced a full blown panic attack. This frightened her tremendously, in part because she believed that she too was having a heart attack. Her family doctor saw her later that day, diagnosed the symptoms as anxiety, reassured her and gave her a limited prescription of diazepam, 5 mg.

However, the initial attack was not an isolated episode; in the ensuing weeks she experienced approximately four attacks per week. This continued to occur even after she was reassured that her father was making a safe recovery. Most attacks were spontaneous (not associated with acute stressful precipitants). They came on rapidly (about 2 minutes from the first sign of symptoms to the height of the attack) and subsided, usually within 5–10 minutes.

Ms. B. was again seen by her physician who ran a battery of tests and concluded that aside from the panic attacks, she was in good health.

Diagnostic Issues: As noted in the previous case, anytime anxiety is seen as a dominant symptom, it is important to rule out medical causes, including substance use/abuse. Ms. B. denied alcohol and illicit drug use, but did admit to drinking 3–4 cups of coffee and at least one diet cola per day. Caffeine rarely causes full blown panic attacks, although it often contributes significantly to generalized anxiety and can lower the threshold for panic attacks. Thus, she was advised to gradually (over a period of 3 weeks) replace coffee and sodas with decaffeinated beverages. The gradual reduction in caffeine was done to reduce the likelihood of caffeine withdrawal (a problem frequently seen with abrupt discontinuation). In Ms. B.'s case the reduction in caffeine did reduce some generalized anxiety and improved her ability to fall asleep at night. However, the frequency of panic attacks was relatively unchanged. It is also worth noting that the prn use of 5 mg. diazepam did little to ward off her periodic attacks.

As in the last case, the clinician asked detailed questions to assess for the presence of depression. In Ms. B's case, she was beginning to feel quite discouraged and sad. She also experienced a good deal of pessimistic thinking, low self-esteem and fatigue. But other signs of a major depression were absent.

The diagnostic impression is one of panic disorder with associated mild depressive symptoms.

Initial Medication Treatment Issues and Decisions: The clinician decided to use a two-pronged approach: a) she was started on the antidepressant paroxetine, and b) referral to a psychotherapist who specialized in behavioral treatment. She had developed some phobias about leaving her house and this would be the target for behavioral treatment once panic symptoms were eliminated or reduced.

Course of Treatment: The initial dose of paroxetine was 20 mg. q.h.s., which she tolerated well. On day 7 the dose was increased to 30 mg. q.h.s., however, the next day she experienced two panic attacks. An *increase* in anxiety and panic symptoms often occurs during the first 2–3 weeks of treatment with antidepressants. Thus, although this was a complication, it was not completely unexpected. The clinician then decided to add alprazolam 1.0 mg. t.i.d. to the 30 mg. of paroxetine (common and often successful strategy). The panic attacks subsided; Ms. B. only experienced two attacks during the next week and these were less intense than prior attacks.

The clinician continued to increase the paroxetine dose to a level of 40 mg. q.h.s. and after three weeks reduced the dose of alprazolam to 0.5 mg. t.i.d. (for one week) followed by a further reduction (0.25 mg. t.i.d.). Since the increase in paroxetine, Ms. B. has only experienced two additional minor attacks (sometimes referred to as limited symptom attacks).

By week five the alprazolam was discontinued altogether. However, the next day Ms. B. experienced her first full blown attack in several weeks. Several questions must be asked at this point:

- Were there any new or increased psychosocial stressors?
- Did she consume alcohol or caffeine within the past day?

In Ms. B.'s case, there were no new or increased stressors, no alcohol or caffeine use, and she did take her medications as prescribed. The most likely hypothesis was the low dose of alprazolam was, in fact, instrumental in warding off panic attacks.

The clinician reinstated the alprazolam at 0.25 mg. t.i.d. and continued the paroxetine dose at 40 mg. q.h.s. No further attacks occurred during the next week. Then the alprazolam was again discontinued. Ms. B. remained stable over the next two weeks, with only one limited symptom attack. She was also told she could take one 0.25 mg. alprazolam as needed for situational anxiety (which she did 2–3 times per week over the next two months).

With panic symptoms well controlled, the behavior therapist began using graded exposure techniques with Ms. B. to help her overcome her phobia. In addition she began to explore her feelings related to her father's illness and what she identified as "my problems growing up and separating from my parents." She continued to deal with these psychological issues in psychotherapy, long after all panic and phobic symptoms disappeared.

Nine months after starting treatment, her physician initiated a gradual reduction of the paroxetine. However, five days after taking a dose of 30 mg. q.h.s., Ms. B. had another panic attack. It was necessary to resume the 40 mg. q.h.s. dose. Four months later a gradual discontinuation trial was successful.

Psychotropic medication treatment is very effective with panic disorders, but almost always requires concurrent psychotherapy and/or behavior therapy.

CASE F: A Case of Acute Schizophrenia

Background and Presenting Problems: Mr. P. is a 22 year-old, unmarried janitor who comes to the clinic complaining of "insomnia." He has been experiencing initial insomnia, restless sleep, and "bad dreams" during the past month. He is quite thin and has marginal personal hygiene, but otherwise is in good health. He reports some alcohol use but denies abuse of illicit drugs. He smokes three packs of cigarettes per day and drinks "a lot of coffee."

In addition to his reported problems, upon clinical evaluation you discover that he has been hearing voices over the past few weeks. The voices generally mumble unintelligible things to him, and on occasion he will hear them say, "you are a loser." He is not especially concerned about the voices, but does worry a lot about buses that pass his apartment. "The way they slow down right by my apartment is weird . . . I think they are sent there to watch me." Beyond this vague description of the activity of buses, he can offer little additional elaboration. Mr. P. also appears to be quite anxious and somewhat agitated.

Mr. P. graduated from high school with a C+ average. He has always been a loner, and his only real human connections are with his immediate family, who live nearby. There is no prior history of psychiatric treatment. He strikes you as a rather shallow and empty man.

Diagnostic Issues: The history and evolution of his symptoms suggest the picture of acute psychosis (likely schizophrenia, although because of the absence of prior florid psychotic symptoms, initially this is best seen as schizophreniform disorder). He is evaluated medically to rule out disorders that may cause psychosis (none are found) and you learn that he takes no prescription medications. There have been no acute psychosocial stressors precipitating his slip into psychosis.

Initial Medication Treatment Issues and Decisions: The treatment of choice for schizophrenia are antipsychotics; Mr. P. is prescribed olanzapine 2.5 mg. b.i.d.

Scenario One: Mr. P. tolerates the olanzapine and on day 4 you increase the dose to 5 mg. b.i.d. Within a week he reports to you that he is sleeping better, and he appears somewhat less anxious. However, unrealistic thinking, auditory hallucinations and inadequate personal hygiene continue.

After 5 weeks of treatment, Mr. P. reports that the voices have stopped. Two weeks later, when again questioned about the buses, he states, "Oh, they aren't bothering me . . . I haven't paid much attention to them lately." Hygiene has improved a bit. He appears to be significantly less anxious, although he remains socially isolated and emotionally empty.

Treatment is continued for an additional ten months and then the haloperidol is gradually reduced over a period of six weeks. Mr. P. is stable and not psychotic. Followup appointments are scheduled on a once-a-month basis, and he is monitored closely, especially because his disorder is notoriously recurring.

Scenario Two: Mr. P. is treated with haloperidol, 3 mg. b.i.d. However, within the first week of treatment he develops side effects: a mild tremor and feelings of increased restlessness (probably akathisia). He is prescribed the anticholinergic benzotropine, 5 mg. q.d., and within a few days the side effects disappear. He continues on the benzotropine until the haloperidol is phased out ten months later.

Scenario Three: Mr. P. does not respond to the 6 mg. q.d. of haloperidol and develops considerable side effect problems: marked restlessness, dystonias and flat affect. The coadministration of benzotropine reduces side effects somewhat, but after three weeks of treatment, there are no noticeable changes in his psychotic symptoms. The haloperidol is increased, first to 8 mg. q.d., and a week later to 10 mg. q.d. He is now sleeping somewhat better, but extrapyramidal symptoms have increased and are only partially responding to benzotropine. You are concerned both by the lack of response to haloperidol and the concern that he will (due to unpleasant side effects) either drop out of treatment or fail to comply with the medication treatment.

The decision is made to discontinue the haloperidol and benzotropine, and begin treating Mr. P. with risperidone 2 mg. b.i.d. He tolerates this medication well and within a week appears to be more calm. At day 14, hallucinations and delusional thinking continue, so the dose of risperidone is increased to 3 mg. b.i.d. By day 22, Mr. P. reports, "the voices have stopped," and during the following two weeks his thinking gradually becomes more rational and realistic. By the seventh week of treatment, Mr. P. appears to be somewhat more spontaneous and there is a noticeable change in personal hygiene. He is showing a good response to the new medication, and continues to take it at the 3 mg. b.i.d. dose for ten months. At that time you gradually reduce the dose.

In each scenario the clinician had the patient sign an informed consent for treatment and remained alert to the emergence of any abnormal movements that might signal the onset of tardive dyskinesia. Under the best of circumstances, Mr. P. will continue to be at risk for relapse, although since it was his first psychotic episode, it was reasonable to conduct a trial without medications about one year following his initial treatment. It is wise to also talk with the patient and (if appropriate) with his family about warning signs of possible relapse, so that should this occur, antipsychotic medications can be started immediately.

Appendix A
History and Personal Data Questionnaire

Date: _____

Name: _____ Date of birth: _____ Age: _____

Main reason for seeking help at this time: _____

_____

_____

Current Problems or Symptoms

Please read each item below and determine which statement is true for you. Then, place an "**X**" in the appropriate box to indicate how often you feel the statement applies to you *during the past month or since your last visit.*

EXAMPLE **Be sure to rate every item.**	None or a little of the time	Some of the time	Most or all of the time
1. I feel sad		X	

	DURING THE PAST MONTH OR SINCE LAST VISIT	None or a little of the time	Some of the time	Most or all of the time
A	1. Wake up at night in the early morning and unable to return to sleep			
	2. Very restless sleep			
	3. Fatigue or loss of energy			
	4. Decreased sex drive			
	5. Unable to enjoy life; have lost a zest for life			
	6. Have withdrawn from others			
	7. Strong thoughts about suicide			
	8. Loss of appetite			
	9. Memory problem, forgetfulness, poor concentration			
	10. Feel irritable or easily frustrated			
	11. Feelings of sadness or hopelessness			
	12. Sleeping a lot			
B	13. Decreased need for sleep			
	14. Increased sex drive			
	15. Increased energy			
	16. So happy or energetic that people describe me as "manic"			
C	17. Can't get to sleep			

Appendix A
History and Personal Data Questionnaire, Cont'd.

DURING THE PAST MONTH OR SINCE LAST VISIT	None or a little of the time	Some of the time	Most or all of the time
18. Sudden episodes of nervousness or panic			
19. Fear of losing self-control			
20. Palpitations or rapid heart beat			
21. Shortness of breath			
22. Feel tense or anxious all day			
23. Feel very anxious in social situations			
24. Have recurring, troubling , thoughts, images or impulses that I can't get out of my mind			
25. Repetitive behaviors such as excessive hand washing, etc.			
D 26. Feel very confused about my thoughts			
27. Strange or bizarre thoughts			
28. Hallucinations, hear voices, or see things that aren't there			
29. Very peculiar experiences that others do not understand			
E 30. Feel ready to explode			
31. Thoughts about harming someone			
32. Excessive use of alcohol/drugs			
F 33. Unusual eating habits			
34. Weight loss—How much in past month? ____ lbs. Weight gain—How much in past month? ____ lbs. Have you been trying to diet? ____ Yes ____ No			
35. In the past I have tried to cut down on my use of alcohol or other drugs ____ Yes ____ No			

Previous Treatment for Psychological or Emotional Problems

Year	Problem	Therapist/Location	Hospitalization or Medical Treatment

Do You Take Any of the Following Medications?
❏ Antihypertensives (for high blood pressure or migraine headaches)
❏ Steroids   ❏ Hormones   ❏ Tranquilizers

Thank You

Appendix B

SPECIAL CAUTIONS WHEN TAKING MAO INHIBITORS

A Patient Hand-Out

MAO Inhibitors can be very safe and effective antidepressant medications. However, certain foods and drugs must be avoided while taking MAO Inhibitors. Mixing MAO Inhibitors with the following drugs/foods can cause a serious rise in blood pressure.

FOODS TO AVOID

- Cheese (Philadelphia cream cheese and cottage cheese are OK.)
- Chicken liver and beef liver
- Yeast preparations (avoid Brewer's yeast, powdered and caked yeast as sold in health food stores, Bakery yeast is OK.)
- Fava or broad beans
- Herring (pickled or kippered)
- Beer, sherry, ale, red wine, liqueurs
- Canned figs
- Protein extracts (found in some dried soups, soup cubes, and commercial gravies)
- Certain meat products; bologna, salami, pepperoni, Spam

AVOID EXCESSIVE AMOUNTS OF THESE FOODS

- Yogurt and/or sour cream
- Ripe avacados and guacamole
- Chocolate and/or caffeine
- White wine and liquors

MEDICATIONS TO AVOID

- Stimulant drugs (amphetamines, dexadrine, benzedine, methedrine, methylphenidate)
- Diet pills
- Cocaine, "crack"
- Cold preparations, including over-the-counter products which contain decongestants (e.g., Sudafed, Contac, etc.). Antihistamines and aspirin are OK.

- Nasal sprays
- Adrenalin (Make sure that your dentist knows you are taking MAO Inhibitors because many local anesthetics contain adrenalin.)
- Please talk with your physician before taking any new medications (prescription or over-the-counter.)

SYMPTOMS OF DRUG FOOD INTERACTION

While taking MAO Inhibitors, if you ever experience the following symptoms, please contact your physician or an emergency room immediately.

- Severe headache
- Excessive perspiration
- Lightheadedness
- Vomiting
- Increased heart rate

I have read and understand the above precautions.

Patient's Name _____ Date _____

Signature

References

American Psychiatric Association (1987) *Diagnostic and Statistical Manual of Mental Disorders-III-Revised* (DSM-IIIR). APA, Washington, DC.

Baldessarini, R. J. and Cole J. O. (1988) "Chemotherapy" in *The New Harvard Guide to Psychiatry,* edited by A. M. Nicholi, Harvard University Press, Cambridge, Mass.

Depression in Primary Care: Treatment of Major Depression. (1993) Rockville, MD, U.S. Department of Health and Human Services, AHCPR Pub. No. 93-0551.

Goldberg, Stephen (1999) *The Four-Minute Neurologic Exam,* MedMaster, Inc., Miami.

Katon, W. (1994) *Panic Disorder in the Medical Setting* Rockville, MD, U.S. Department of Health and Human Services, NIH Pub. No. 94-3482.

Klein, D. (1995) *Dysthymia and Atypical Depression* U.S. Psychiatric and Mental Health Congress.

Kutcher, S. (2002) *Practical Child and Adolescent Psychopharmacology,* Cambridge University Press.

Maxmen, J. and Ward, N. (1995) *Psychotropic Drugs: Fast Facts* (Second edition) W. W. Norton and Company, New York.

Nicholi, A. M. (ed.) (1988) *The New Harvard Guide to Psychiatry,* Harvard University Press, Cambridge Mass.

Pearlman, C. A. (1986) "Neuroleptic malignant syndrome: A review of the literature." *Journal of Clinical Psychopharmacology,* 6:257–273.

Practice Guideline for Major Depressive Disorder in Adults (1993) American Psychiatric Association, Washington, D.C.

Preston, J., Lucas, J., and O'Neal, J. (1995) *Understanding Psychiatric Medications in the Treatment of Chemical Dependency and Dual Diagnosis.* Charles C. Thomas, Springfield, Ill.

Preston, J. D., O'Neal, J. H. and Talaga, M. C. (2002) *Handbook of Clinical Psychopharmacology for Therapists.* New Harbinger Publications, Oakland, CA.

Rush, A. John (1997) *Strategies and Tactics in the Treatment of Mood Disorders.* American Psychiatric Press, Washington, D.C.

Texas Medication Algorithm Project: *http://asedillo.home.texas.net/tmap.htm*

Unlenhuth E. H. DeWit, H., Balter, M. B., Johanson, C. E. and Mellinger, G. D. (1988) "Risks and benefits of long term benzodiazepine use." *Journal of Clinical Psychopharmacology,* 8:161–167.

Index